MW01258773

# TABLE OF CONTENTS

# Secret Key #1 - Time is Your Greatest Enemy

## *Pace Yourself*

Wear a watch. At the beginning of the test, check the time (or start a chronometer on your watch to count the minutes), and check the time after every few questions to make sure you are "on schedule."

If you are forced to speed up, do it efficiently. Usually one or more answer choices can be eliminated without too much difficulty. Above all, don't panic. Don't speed up and just begin guessing at random choices. By pacing yourself, and continually monitoring your progress against your watch, you will always know exactly how far ahead or behind you are with your available time. If you find that you are one minute behind on the test, don't skip one question without spending any time on it, just to catch back up. Take 15 fewer seconds on the next four questions, and after four questions you'll have caught back up. Once you catch back up, you can continue working each problem at your normal pace.

Furthermore, don't dwell on the problems that you were rushed on. If a problem was taking up too much time and you made a hurried guess, it must be difficult. The difficult questions are the ones you are most likely to miss anyway, so it isn't a big loss. It is better to end with more time than you need than to run out of time.

Lastly, sometimes it is beneficial to slow down if you are constantly getting ahead of time. You are always more likely to catch a careless mistake by working more slowly than quickly, and among very high-scoring test takers (those who are likely to have lots of time left over), careless errors affect the score more than mastery of material.

# Secret Key #2 - Guessing is not Guesswork

You probably know that guessing is a good idea - unlike other standardized tests, there is no penalty for getting a wrong answer. Even if you have no idea about a question, you still have a 20-25% chance of getting it right.

Most test takers do not understand the impact that proper guessing can have on their score. Unless you score extremely high, guessing will significantly contribute to your final score.

## Monkeys Take the Test

What most test takers don't realize is that to insure that 20-25% chance, you have to guess randomly. If you put 20 monkeys in a room to take this test, assuming they answered once per question and behaved themselves, on average they would get 20-25% of the questions correct. Put 20 test takers in the room, and the average will be much lower among guessed questions. Why?

1. The test writers intentionally writes deceptive answer choices that "look" right. A test taker has no idea about a question, so picks the "best looking" answer, which is often wrong. The monkey has no idea what looks good and what doesn't, so will consistently be lucky about 20-25% of the time.

2. Test takers will eliminate answer choices from the guessing pool based on a hunch or intuition. Simple but correct answers often get excluded, leaving a 0% chance of being correct. The monkey has no clue, and often gets lucky with the best choice.

This is why the process of elimination endorsed by most test courses is flawed and detrimental to your performance- test takers don't guess, they make an ignorant stab in the dark that is usually worse than random.

## $5 Challenge

Let me introduce one of the most valuable ideas of this course- the $5 challenge:

*You only mark your "best guess" if you are willing to bet $5 on it.*

*You only eliminate choices from guessing if you are willing to bet $5 on it.*

Why $5? Five dollars is an amount of money that is small yet not insignificant, and can really add up fast (20 questions could cost you $100). Likewise, each answer choice on one question of the test will have a small impact on your overall score, but it can really add up to a lot of points in the end.

The process of elimination IS valuable. The following shows your chance of guessing it right:

| If you eliminate wrong answer choices until only this many remain: | 1 | 2 | 3 |
|---|---|---|---|
| Chance of getting it correct: | 100% | 50% | 33% |

However, if you accidentally eliminate the right answer or go on a hunch for an incorrect answer, your chances drop dramatically: to 0%. By guessing among all the answer choices, you are GUARANTEED to have a shot at the right answer.

That's why the $5 test is so valuable- if you give up the advantage and safety of a pure guess, it had better be worth the risk.

What we still haven't covered is how to be sure that whatever guess you make is truly random. Here's the easiest way:

*Always pick the first answer choice among those remaining.*

Such a technique means that you have decided, **before you see a single test question**, exactly how you are going to guess- and since the order of choices tells you nothing about which one is correct, this guessing technique is perfectly random.

This section is not meant to scare you away from making educated guesses or eliminating choices- you just need to define when a choice is worth eliminating. The $5 test, along with a pre-defined random guessing strategy, is the best way to make sure you reap all of the benefits of guessing.

# Secret Key #3 - Practice Smarter, Not Harder

Many test takers delay the test preparation process because they dread the awful amounts of practice time they think necessary to succeed on the test. We have refined an effective method that will take you only a fraction of the time.

There are a number of "obstacles" in your way to succeed. Among these are answering questions, finishing in time, and mastering test-taking strategies. All must be executed on the day of the test at peak performance, or your score will suffer. The test is a mental marathon that has a large impact on your future.

Just like a marathon runner, it is important to work your way up to the full challenge. So first you just worry about questions, and then time, and finally strategy:

## *Success Strategy*

1. Find a good source for practice tests.
2. If you are willing to make a larger time investment, consider using more than one study guide- often the different approaches of multiple authors will help you "get" difficult concepts.
3. Take a practice test with no time constraints, with all study helps "open book." Take your time with questions and focus on applying strategies.
4. Take a practice test with time constraints, with all guides "open book."
5. Take a final practice test with no open material and time limits

If you have time to take more practice tests, just repeat step 5. By gradually exposing yourself to the full rigors of the test environment, you will condition your mind to the stress of test day and maximize your success.

# Secret Key #4 - Prepare, Don't Procrastinate

Let me state an obvious fact: if you take the test three times, you will get three different scores. This is due to the way you feel on test day, the level of preparedness you have, and, despite the test writers' claims to the contrary, some tests WILL be easier for you than others.

Since your future depends so much on your score, you should maximize your chances of success. In order to maximize the likelihood of success, you've got to prepare in advance. This means taking practice tests and spending time learning the information and test taking strategies you will need to succeed.

Never take the test as a "practice" test, expecting that you can just take it again if you need to. Feel free to take sample tests on your own, but when you go to take the official test, be prepared, be focused, and do your best the first time!

# Secret Key #5 - Test Yourself

Everyone knows that time is money. There is no need to spend too much of your time or too little of your time preparing for the test. You should only spend as much of your precious time preparing as is necessary for you to get the score you need.

Once you have taken a practice test under real conditions of time constraints, then you will know if you are ready for the test or not.

If you have scored extremely high the first time that you take the practice test, then there is not much point in spending countless hours studying. You are already there.

Benchmark your abilities by retaking practice tests and seeing how much you have improved. Once you score high enough to guarantee success, then you are ready.

If you have scored well below where you need, then knuckle down and begin studying in earnest. Check your improvement regularly through the use of practice tests under real conditions. Above all, don't worry, panic, or give up. The key is perseverance!

Then, when you go to take the test, remain confident and remember how well you did on the practice tests. If you can score high enough on a practice test, then you can do the same on the real thing.

# General Strategies

The most important thing you can do is to ignore your fears and jump into the test immediately- do not be overwhelmed by any strange-sounding terms. You have to jump into the test like jumping into a pool- all at once is the easiest way.

## Make Predictions

As you read and understand the question, try to guess what the answer will be. Remember that several of the answer choices are wrong, and once you begin reading them, your mind will immediately become cluttered with answer choices designed to throw you off. Your mind is typically the most focused immediately after you have read the question and digested its contents. If you can, try to predict what the correct answer will be. You may be surprised at what you can predict.

Quickly scan the choices and see if your prediction is in the listed answer choices. If it is, then you can be quite confident that you have the right answer. It still won't hurt to check the other answer choices, but most of the time, you've got it!

## Answer the Question

It may seem obvious to only pick answer choices that answer the question, but the test writers can create some excellent answer choices that are wrong. Don't pick an answer just because it sounds right, or you believe it to be true. It MUST answer the question. Once you've made your selection, always go back and check it against the question and make sure that you didn't misread the question, and the answer choice does answer the question posed.

## Benchmark

After you read the first answer choice, decide if you think it sounds correct or not. If it doesn't, move on to the next answer choice. If it does, mentally mark that answer choice. This doesn't mean that you've definitely selected it as your answer choice, it just means that it's the best you've seen thus far. Go ahead and read the next choice. If the next choice is worse than the one you've already selected, keep going to the next answer choice. If the next choice is better than the choice you've already selected, mentally mark the new answer choice as your best guess.

The first answer choice that you select becomes your standard. Every other answer choice must be benchmarked against that standard. That choice is correct until proven otherwise by another answer choice beating it out. Once you've decided that no other answer choice seems as good, do one final check to ensure that your answer choice answers the question posed.

## Valid Information

Don't discount any of the information provided in the question. Every piece of information may be necessary to determine the correct answer. None of the information in the question is there to throw you off (while the answer choices will certainly have information to throw you off). If two seemingly unrelated topics are discussed, don't ignore either. You can be confident there is a relationship, or it wouldn't be included in the question, and you are probably going to have to determine what is that relationship to find the answer.

## Avoid "Fact Traps"

Don't get distracted by a choice that is factually true. Your search is for the answer that answers the question. Stay focused and don't fall for an answer that is true but incorrect. Always go back to the question and make sure you're choosing an answer that actually answers the question and is not just a true statement. An answer can be factually correct, but it MUST answer the question asked. Additionally, two answers can both be seemingly correct, so be sure to read all of the answer choices, and make sure that you get the one that BEST answers the question.

## Milk the Question

Some of the questions may throw you completely off. They might deal with a subject you have not been exposed to, or one that you haven't reviewed in years. While your lack of knowledge about the subject will be a hindrance, the question itself can give you many clues that will help you find the correct answer. Read the question carefully and look for clues. Watch particularly for adjectives and nouns describing difficult terms or words that you don't recognize. Regardless of if you completely understand a word or not, replacing it with a synonym either provided or one you more familiar with may help you to understand what the questions are asking. Rather than wracking your mind about specific detailed information concerning a difficult term or word, try to use mental substitutes that are easier to understand.

## The Trap of Familiarity

Don't just choose a word because you recognize it. On difficult questions, you may not recognize a number of words in the answer choices. The test writers don't put "make-believe" words on the test; so don't think that just because you only recognize all the words in one answer choice means that answer choice must be correct. If you only recognize words in one answer choice, then focus on that one. Is it correct? Try your best to determine if it is correct. If it is, that is great, but if it doesn't, eliminate it. Each word and answer choice you eliminate increases your chances of getting the question correct, even if you then have to guess among the unfamiliar choices.

## Eliminate Answers

Eliminate choices as soon as you realize they are wrong. But be careful! Make sure you consider all of the possible answer choices. Just because one appears right, doesn't mean that the next one won't be even better! The test writers will usually put more than one good answer choice for every question, so read all of them. Don't worry if you are stuck between two that seem right. By getting down to just two remaining possible choices, your odds are now 50/50. Rather than wasting too much time, play the odds. You are guessing, but guessing wisely, because you've been able to knock out some of the answer choices that you know are wrong. If you are eliminating choices and realize that the last answer choice you are left with is also obviously wrong, don't panic. Start over and consider each choice again. There may easily be something that you missed the first time and will realize on the second pass.

## Tough Questions

If you are stumped on a problem or it appears too hard or too difficult, don't waste time. Move on! Remember though, if you can quickly check for obviously incorrect answer choices, your chances of guessing correctly are greatly improved. Before you completely give up, at least try to knock out a couple of possible answers. Eliminate what you can and then guess at the remaining answer choices before moving on.

## Brainstorm

If you get stuck on a difficult question, spend a few seconds quickly brainstorming. Run through the complete list of possible answer choices. Look at each choice and ask yourself, "Could this answer the question satisfactorily?" Go through each answer choice and consider it independently of the other. By systematically going through all possibilities, you may find something that you would otherwise overlook. Remember that when you get stuck, it's important to try to keep moving.

## Read Carefully

Understand the problem. Read the question and answer choices carefully. Don't miss the question because you misread the terms. You have plenty of time to read each question thoroughly and make sure you understand what is being asked. Yet a happy medium must be attained, so don't waste too much time. You must read carefully, but efficiently.

## Face Value

When in doubt, use common sense. Always accept the situation in the problem at face value. Don't read too much into it. These problems will not require you to make huge leaps of logic. The test writers aren't trying to throw you off with a cheap trick. If you have to go beyond creativity and make a leap of logic in order to have an answer choice answer the question, then you should look at the other answer choices. Don't overcomplicate the problem by creating theoretical relationships or explanations that will warp time or space. These are normal problems rooted in reality. It's just that the applicable relationship or explanation may not be readily apparent and you have to figure things out. Use your common sense to interpret anything that isn't clear.

## Prefixes

If you're having trouble with a word in the question or answer choices, try dissecting it. Take advantage of every clue that the word might include. Prefixes and suffixes can be a huge help. Usually they allow you to determine a basic meaning. Pre- means before, post- means after, pro - is positive, de- is negative. From these prefixes and suffixes, you can get an idea of the general meaning of the word and try to put it into context. Beware though of any traps. Just because con is the opposite of pro, doesn't necessarily mean congress is the opposite of progress!

## Hedge Phrases

Watch out for critical "hedge" phrases, such as likely, may, can, will often, sometimes, often, almost, mostly, usually, generally, rarely, sometimes. Question writers insert these hedge phrases to cover every possibility. Often an answer choice will be wrong simply because it leaves no room for exception. Avoid answer choices that have definitive words like "exactly," and "always".

## Switchback Words

Stay alert for "switchbacks". These are the words and phrases frequently used to alert you to shifts in thought. The most common switchback word is "but". Others include although, however, nevertheless, on the other hand, even though, while, in spite of, despite, regardless of.

## New Information

Correct answer choices will rarely have completely new information included. Answer choices typically are straightforward reflections of the material asked about and will directly relate to the question. If a new piece of information is included in an answer choice that doesn't even seem to relate to the topic being asked about, then that answer choice is likely incorrect. All of the information needed to answer the question is usually provided for you, and so you should not have to make guesses that are unsupported or choose answer choices that require unknown information that cannot be reasoned on its own.

## Time Management

On technical questions, don't get lost on the technical terms. Don't spend too much time on any one question. If you don't know what a term means, then since you don't have a dictionary, odds are you aren't going to get much further. You should immediately recognize terms as whether or not you know them. If you don't, work with the other clues that you have, the other answer choices and terms provided, but don't waste too much time trying to figure out a difficult term.

## Contextual Clues

Look for contextual clues. An answer can be right but not correct. The contextual clues will help you find the answer that is most right and is correct. Understand the context in which a phrase or statement is made. This will help you make important distinctions.

## Don't Panic

Panicking will not answer any questions for you. Therefore, it isn't helpful. When you first see the question, if your mind goes blank, take a deep breath. Force yourself to mechanically go through the steps of solving the problem and using the strategies you've learned.

## Pace Yourself

Don't get clock fever. It's easy to be overwhelmed when you're looking at a page full of questions, your mind is full of random thoughts and feeling confused, and the clock is ticking down faster than you would like. Calm down and maintain the pace that you have set for yourself. As long as you are on track by monitoring your pace, you are guaranteed to have enough time for yourself. When you get to the last few minutes of the test, it may seem like you won't have enough time left, but if you only have as many questions as you should have left at that point, then you're right on track!

## Answer Selection

The best way to pick an answer choice is to eliminate all of those that are wrong, until only one is left and confirm that is the correct answer. Sometimes though, an answer choice may immediately look right. Be careful! Take a second to make sure that the other choices are not equally obvious. Don't make a hasty mistake. There are only two times that you should stop before checking other answers. First is when you are positive that the answer choice you have selected is correct. Second is when time is almost out and you have to make a quick guess!

## Check Your Work

Since you will probably not know every term listed and the answer to every question, it is important that you get credit for the ones that you do know. Don't miss any questions through careless mistakes. If at all possible, try to take a second to look back over your answer selection and make sure you've selected the correct answer choice and haven't made a costly careless mistake (such as marking an answer choice that you didn't mean to mark). This quick double check should more than pay for itself in caught mistakes for the time it costs.

## Beware of Directly Quoted Answers

Sometimes an answer choice will repeat word for word a portion of the question or reference section. However, beware of such exact duplication – it may be a trap! More than likely, the correct choice will paraphrase or summarize a point, rather than being exactly the same wording.

## Slang

Scientific sounding answers are better than slang ones. An answer choice that begins "To compare the outcomes..." is much more likely to be correct than one that begins "Because some people insisted..."

## Extreme Statements

Avoid wild answers that throw out highly controversial ideas that are proclaimed as established fact. An answer choice that states the "process should used in certain situations, if..." is much more likely to be correct than one that states the "process should be discontinued completely." The first is a calm rational statement and doesn't even make a definitive, uncompromising stance, using a hedge word "if" to provide wiggle room, whereas the second choice is a radical idea and far more extreme.

## Answer Choice Families

When you have two or more answer choices that are direct opposites or parallels, one of them is usually the correct answer. For instance, if one answer choice states "x increases" and another answer choice states "x decreases" or "y increases," then those two or three answer choices are very similar in construction and fall into the same family of answer choices. A family of answer choices is when two or three answer choices are very similar in construction, and yet often have a directly opposite meaning. Usually the correct answer choice will be in that family of answer choices. The "odd man out" or answer choice that doesn't seem to fit the parallel construction of the other answer choices is more likely to be incorrect.

# Top 20 Test Taking Tips

1. Carefully follow all the test registration procedures

2. Know the test directions, duration, topics, question types, how many questions

3. Setup a flexible study schedule at least 3-4 weeks before test day

4. Study during the time of day you are most alert, relaxed, and stress free

5. Maximize your learning style; visual learner use visual study aids, auditory learner use auditory study aids

6. Focus on your weakest knowledge base

7. Find a study partner to review with and help clarify questions

8. Practice, practice, practice

9. Get a good night's sleep; don't try to cram the night before the test

10. Eat a well balanced meal

11. Know the exact physical location of the testing site; drive the route to the site prior to test day

12. Bring a set of ear plugs; the testing center could be noisy

13. Wear comfortable, loose fitting, layered clothing to the testing center; prepare for it to be either cold or hot during the test

14. Bring at least 2 current forms of ID to the testing center

15. Arrive to the test early; be prepared to wait and be patient

16. Eliminate the obviously wrong answer choices, then guess the first remaining choice

17. Pace yourself; don't rush, but keep working and move on if you get stuck

18. Maintain a positive attitude even if the test is going poorly

19. Keep your first answer unless you are positive it is wrong

20. Check your work, don't make a careless mistake

# Nutrition Screeningand Diagnosis

**Assessment versus screening**

Nutrition assessment is the determination of the nutritional status of an individual in order to implement appropriate interventions as needed. Nutrition screening is the identification of individuals at risk for compromised nutritional status using a screening tool. The Nutrition Screening Initiative (NSI) was developed in 1991, as a joint effort between the American Dietetic Association (ADA), the American Academy of Family Physicians (AAFP), and the National Council on Aging (NCOA), along with experts and advisors from the fields of health, medicine, aging and nutrition. The NSI was developed because the 1988 Surgeon General's Workshop on Health Promotion and Aging and the Department of Health and Human Services (DHHS) identified the need for nutrition screening. A screening manual and checklist were developed to aide in the identification of geriatric populations with nutritional risk, and those materials were distributed to doctors' offices, senior centers, hospitals, nursing homes, adult daycare programs, nutrition programs for elderly adults, and other healthcare programs.

The Level I screening tool is used after the initial tool identifies individuals who require further nutrition assessment based on results from body mass index calculations, dietary habit evaluation, living situation, and functional status. This tool may be used by many different types of caregivers and may determine the need for further medical, social service or nutritional interventions. A Level II screening must be completed by a specially trained healthcare provider and involves anthropometric assessment, laboratory tests, full evaluation of medication use, social/living situation, eating habits, neurological status, and functional status. Additional screening tools that are specifically directed towards oral health, drug-nutrient interaction and dietary counseling are available as algorithms for initiating nutrition support and for implementing NSI in various clinical settings.

**DETERMINE**

The acronym "DETERMINE" (developed by the Nutrition Screening Initiative) is the basis for the nutritional health checklist, which identifies warning signs for nutritional problems.  The acronym stands for:

- **D**isease
- **E**ating poorly
- **T**ooth loss/mouth pain
- **E**conomic hardship
- **R**educed social contact
- **M**ultiple medicines
- **I**nvoluntary weight loss or gain
- **N**eeds assistance with self-care
- **E**lder years - above age 80

The checklist consists of 10 questions, including the impact of any illnesses on eating, fruit, vegetable and dairy intake, amount of alcohol consumed, social and financial situation, condition of teeth, medication use, and weight changes.

In the "DETERMINE Your Nutritional Health Checklist," disease was included as a warning sign of possible nutritional deficiencies because any type of disease or chronic illness may impact nutritional status.  Many chronic diseases are affected by diet, and the often concurrent presence of depression may also affect nutritional status and appetite.  Eating poorly is included as a warning sign of nutritional problems because under eating and overeating may both adversely affect health and nutrition.  Additionally, if an individual's diet does not include a variety of foods such as fruits, vegetables and dairy products, nutritional status will be impacted.  Alcohol intake may also negatively impact nutritional health.

Tooth loss/ mouth pain is included as a warning sign because oral discomfort affects one's ability to chew, swallow, and taste foods.

The "DETERMINE Your Nutritional Health Checklist," includes economic hardship as a warning sign of nutritional deficiencies because income is often substantially reduced in geriatric populations and this impacts the ability to purchase healthy foods. Reduced social contact is included as a warning sign because as many as a third of all elderly individuals live alone, and this may affect one's desire to eat. Multiple medicines is included as a warning sign because as many as 50% of elderly individuals take more than one medication on a daily basis. As more medications are added to a person's daily regime, side effects, such as changes in appetite, changes in bowel habits, and others, and drug interactions increase.

Involuntary weight loss/gain is included on the "Determine Your Nutritional Health Checklist as a warning sign of poor nutritional health because changes in weight may indicate an underlying medical condition. Also, being overweight or underweight may adversely affect health status. Needs assistance in self-care is included as a warning sign because many elderly adults may have difficulty walking, shopping, buying or cooking food. Elder years above age 80 is included as a warning sign because as age advances, the risk for developing health issues and needing assistance increases, and these individuals need to be identified in a timely manner to address the issues.

## Mini Nutritional Assessment (MNA)

The Mini Nutritional Assessment (MNA) is a screening tool, developed by Nestle, that has been validated for use in the geriatric (older than 65) population to identify malnutrition. The tool asks questions about changes in appetite, weight changes, and ability to move around. Questions are asked about recent life stressors, such as death of a spouse or the onset of newly diagnosed diseases or dementia. Body mass index (BMI), mid-arm circumference and calf circumference are calculated. The individual's living situation and medication use are assessed. The status of the individual's skin is assessed. Consumed meal frequency, daily fluid intake and the variety of foods eaten are noted. The ability of the individual to self-feed is recorded. The tool asks the individual about his/her perception of his/her nutritional status and asks the individual to compare his/her status to that of his/her peers. The total score is tallied, the degree of malnutrition is assessed, and the need for referral to a dietitian is determined.

**Other nutrition screening tools**

Other screening tools available include:
- *Body mass index (BMI):* This is calculated by dividing weight (kg) by squared height (meters $^2$). A normal range BMI falls between 22-27 kg/m$^2$. Values higher or lower than this range may indicate that the patient is obese or underweight.
- *Serum albumin:* Although albumin is affected by a great many factors, using it as a quick screening tool may be a general indicator of possible poor nutrition. Low serum albumin levels have been associated with higher morbidity and mortality.
- *Dietary reference intakes (DRI) and recommended dietary allowances (RDA):* These are reference values used to evaluate dietary intake of healthy individuals.
- *Activities of daily living (ADLs):* This tool measures the ability to perform self-care tasks such as feeding, bathing, etc.

Instrumental activities of daily living (IADLs): Measures the ability of an individual to live independently, including his/her ability to manage money, medication schedules, take care of household, and ability to provide own transportation.

## Changes in body composition

As a person ages, a 2-3% loss of lean body mass per decade may be expected. Lean body mass is the most metabolically active tissue in the body and as it is lost it is replaced by body fat. As the percentage of body fat increases, there is a concurrent decrease in the metabolic rate. A 15-20% decrease in resting metabolic rate may occur throughout the lifespan. The consequences of the decreased metabolic rate include lower energy requirements and the risk of developing obesity-related chronic diseases, such as diabetes. The loss of skeletal muscle in the aging population causes a decrease in muscle strength and may also contribute to an increased risk of developing a chronic disease. The loss of skeletal strength may also cause loss of physical function, which in turn may affect ability to perform activities of daily life (ADL), including the ability to walk with a steady gait.

## Poor oral health

Poor oral health may encompass many factors. This may include decayed teeth, gum disease, missing teeth, absence of dentures or dentures that fit poorly due to changes in weight. The oral cavity may be impacted by teeth in poor condition, which may in turn lead to extreme pain, tenderness and swelling. Oral pain may lead to changes in the consistency of one's diet and avoidance of certain food groups, such as fresh fruits, vegetables, and/or meats. Many elderly individuals experience dry mouth or xerostomia as a result of aging or as a side effect of medications. This may impact the ability to chew and swallow, which may also lead to the avoidance of certain foods. Many elderly people will neglect their oral health and forgo dental treatment. Good oral health contributes to overall physical wellbeing, positive self-image, ability to chew food adequately, and ability to speak effectively.

## Dehydration risk factors

Medication use is a potential cause of dehydration in elderly adults; this risk escalates with the number of medication and becomes prominent in populations taking four or more medications. Diuretic and laxative use and abuse commonly lead to dehydration. Older individuals who have poor appetite, are depressed, have dementia, confusion or other changes in mental status are also at risk. Those that are unable to feed themselves or are dependent on tube feedings or parental nutrition are also at risk. Incontinence, diarrhea, and vomiting may not only cause dehydration but also be the catalyst for self-limitation of foods and fluids. Additionally, elderly adults with multiple medical conditions and/or chronic infections may be at higher risk for dehydration. Chronic illnesses will at some point affect appetite and in turn, fluid intake.

## Taste and smell changes

As the aging process occurs, numerous physical changes in taste and smell may occur that can impact nutritional status. If these changes occur slowly, the individual may gradually adapt to the changes and not notice they are occurring. They may also happen more quickly as a result of illness. In this case, appetite and intake may be affected because there may not be a desire to eat bland tasting food. As the acuity of taste and smell diminishes with the aging process, food will likely become less enjoyable. Often times, changes in sweet and salty sensations occur, which in turn may cause sour and bitter taste sensations to be enhanced. Deficiencies in certain vitamins and minerals such as the B vitamins, vitamin A or zinc may also impact taste.

**Functional assessment** = (ADL's)

*[handwritten: IADL's = ie. driving, Managing finances]*

A functional assessment is a review of an individual's ability to perform basic activities of daily life (ADL). ADLs include the ability to bathe, dress, feed, use the bathroom and control bladder and bowels. It also includes the ability to transfer in and out of bed independently. Impairment in functional status may directly impact nutritional status by hindering one's ability to shop and purchase food, to prepare food, and to feed oneself. Instrumental activities of daily life (IADL) may also be assessed; and these activities include more difficult skills such as driving, shopping and managing finances. A person may be able to perform various degrees of ADLs and IADLs, such as requiring minor assistance with shopping but able to prepare simple, healthy meals. Or a person may need complete assistance with obtaining food and preparing meals but is able to feed oneself and complete basic cleanup. Thus an entire functional assessment should be performed.

**Factors affecting cognitive function**

Vitamin and mineral deficiencies, such as deficiencies of folate, vitamin B12, vitamin B6, vitamin C, vitamin E and beta-carotene may adversely affect cognitive function. Other changes in cognitive function may be due to a decrease in neurotransmitters, a diminished ability of nerves to conduct properly, memory loss or the development of certain forms of senile dementia, such as Alzheimer's disease. The progression of dementia often results in unexplained weight loss (the etiology of which is unknown). Depression may result from decreases in neurotransmitters or may develop as a result of deteriorating health status, decline in functional status, and loss of family members. Other contributing factors to depression include financial concerns, living alone without frequent social interactions or fear. Depression may lead to changes in weight, poor appetite, impaired digestion, changes in energy levels or changes in dietary habits thus resulting in compromised nutritional status or malnutrition.

**Socioeconomic factors**

Financial resources have a large impact on ability to purchase nutritious foods. Older individuals are often on a fixed income. As the cost of living increases, there may not be a concurrent increase in income leaving less money available for food. Some individuals have adequate financial resources for buying food but may lack availability of fresh produce or meats to purchase. In this situation, foods higher in calories, fat or carbohydrate content may be inappropriately substituted. One's educational level also has impacts nutrition--higher levels of education have been linked with improved nutritional status. The individual's living situation may have an impact on nutritional status and the living situation is determined in part to financial resources. For elderly individuals who live in their own home but require assistance with meals, various options are available. These options include home delivered meals, congregate meals, dining out, or assistance with home health aides. Older individuals who are not able to live at home have various options including retirement homes, assisted living facilities, and skilled care facilities, depending upon financial resources.

**Physiologic changes**

As the aging process evolves, a decrease in height is to be expected. This is due to changes in the vertebrae and changes in posture due to osteoporosis. The decrease in height may range from 0.5-1.5 cm per ten years. As men enter their forties and women enter their fifties, changes in body composition begin to occur. The amount of lean body mass decreases while fat stores increase. This increased fat often accumulates around organs. The amount of subcutaneous fat on extremities also decreases while the amount of fat around the abdominal area increases. Abdominal fat may increase the risk for metabolic syndrome, which includes high blood pressure, hyperlipidemia, and insulin resistance.

**Nutrition Care Process**

<u>First step</u>

The purpose of nutrition assessment is to gather appropriate data in order to determine any existing nutritional issues. This may include an initial assessment or a reassessment. Data may be obtained from medical records; the initial referral; an interview with the individual, family or caregiver; or various types of reports, such as statistical data or epidemiological studies. Data collected includes a diet history or a report detailing nutrient intake of an individual, height, weight, lab data, past medical history, and physical and clinical conditions or issues that may impact nutritional status. Functional status, including social, psychological, cognitive and emotional issues, is also important to note.

The factors involved in a nutritional assessment include evaluation of data and determination of impact on nutritional risk. This includes a review of nutrient intake to determine effects on nutritional risk as it applies to the current clinical condition. It involves the evaluation of the current condition and other diseases that may have nutritional consequence. Psychological, social, and functional issues are assessed to determine effects on access to food, preparation of meals, mobility issues and disease status. The ability to learn and change must be evaluated.

When performing a nutritional assessment the register dietician (RD) must be able to think critically in order to identify potential red-flags, assess body language, effectively collect appropriate date, use the appropriate assessment tools, and apply applicable data. The RD should be able to organize the data in an effective way and know when additional help is needed.

Second step

Nutrition diagnosis is when nutritional issues or potential issues are identified by a registered dietician (RD) with the purpose of establishing goals and interventions to address each issue. The fist component of nutrition diagnosis is identifying the problem or diagnostic label. This is a statement briefly describing the issue using a qualifier such as impaired, increased, or potential for. The second step is identifying etiology or cause and contributing factors to diagnosis. Any factor that relates to the issue, such as social, psychological and environmental factors, should be mentioned as should causes of the problem. The person(s) responsible for addressing the nutritional issue must also be identified in this step. The etiology is linked to the problem using the words "related to." The third step is identification of signs/symptoms. These are the defining characteristics that provide proof of the existence of a nutrition related problem. Signs/symptoms are linked to the etiology using the words "as evidenced by." If only a risk for possible illness is identified, the signs/symptoms are not yet identifiable.

Nutrition diagnostic statements should be brief and succinct, specific to the individual and related to the actual problem. The diagnostic statement should be accurately presented using data that was obtained reliably. This should be written in a PES format – problem, etiology, and signs/symptoms – or just PE if the problem is a risk. Nutrition diagnoses should be ranked in order of importance. The American Dietetic Association has developed a list of nutrition diagnostic terminology to be used for documentation purposes. This list can be found on the ADA website. Examples of nutrition diagnostic statements are as follows:

- Inadequate energy intake, related to insufficient access to food, as evidenced by lack of food in home.

- Inconsistent carbohydrate intake related to poor meal planning as evidenced by blood glucose instability.
- Swallowing difficulty related to recent cerebrovascular accident (CVA) as evidenced by abnormal modified barium swallow.

Potential for weight gain related to recent hip surgery and decreased physical activity.

## Third step

The nutrition intervention step consists of formulating a plan to address the issues identified in the nutrition diagnosis. This step is the foundation for the development of outcome measures and evaluation. The nutrition intervention must be based on science and evidence-based research (if available). Registered dieticians must work in conjunction with the individual, family or caregiver and other professionals to plan and develop the most appropriate intervention plan in order to address the diagnosis. Goals should be objective and measurable. Action steps should be chosen such that the problem is effectively addressed and recommendations mirror current research and standard recommendations. The intervention should be unique to the individual and based on his/her medical history and diagnosis. The implementation phase is when the plan is communicated and put into action. Data should be collected and the plan modified as needed.

## Critical thinking skills

Critical thinking skills are essential to the nutrition diagnosis and intervention phases. Registered dieticians (RD) must train themselves to be open-minded and should be able to reason with patients in order to impart the consequences of continuing/discontinuing lifestyle behaviors. RDs should also be able to review data in order to determine interrelationships with possible reasons for nutritional insufficiencies. The ability to prioritize and set goals is essential. Additionally, an RD should be well-connected to other professionals and know when to seek referrals to and advice from those professionals. Moreover, RDs must be able to match strategies for addressing nutrition diagnosis with the individual's ability to learn and readiness to change. These are skills essential to RDs, and dietary professionals should continue to improve these skills.

Nutrition intervention documentation

Quality documentation is an important part of the entire nutrition care process. Documentation in the nutrition intervention phase should include date and time, the predetermined goals for treatment and the expected outcomes. It should also include individualized recommendations, including any changes in the plan and the reason(s) for those changes. The individual's response to the intervention should be noted. Any additional referrals provided to the individual or additional resources that were used should be documented. The plan for follow-up should also be documented along with the expected frequency of care. If the individual is being discharged from care, supporting rationale should be included.

# Nutrition Data Gathering

**Height**

Most predictive equations for determining appropriate body weight or lean body mass require the use of height. It is very difficult to obtain an accurate height as an individual ages and the spine begins to compress. Spinal ailments such as osteoporosis, curvature of the spine or legs that bow, will prevent an accurate measurement.

To measure height in older individuals who are able to stand, shoes should be removed and light clothing worn. The individual should be on a flat surface and stand upright with heels close together and arms by the side. The head should be positioned so the line of vision is perpendicular to the body. A headboard should be lowered as the individual takes a deep breath. The measurement should be taken to the nearest 0.1 cm. The process should be repeated to ensure accuracy.

<u>Use of arm length measurements</u>

Arm span (also called total arm length), the length of the fully extend arms from fingertips to opposite fingertips, may be used to measure height when necessary. Arm span has been correlated with the maximal height reached by an adult before any height changes began to take place. Studies have shown that arm span does not change at the same rate that height does. However, individuals with arthritis or certain spinal ailment, such as kyphosis or osteoporosis, cannot be accurately measured this way. It is important to note that total arm length may differ between individuals of the same height; therefore, this method is not recognized as a standard measurement.

<u>Alternative methods</u>

Self-reported height may be off by 2 cm or more. Alternate methods for determining height are needed especially for individuals who are not able to stand upright. One method is knee height measurements, which measures from the top of the knee to the bottom of the foot using calipers. This information is then applied to an equation and nomogram to calculate the total height. Another method used for individuals with severe deformities or contractures is segmental height. Individual measurements are taken of each segment of the body from one bony prominence to the next. The sum of those measures is then calculated.

**Weight**

If possible, standardized procedures should always be followed to ensure consistent measurements. Individuals should be weighed without shoes and in light clothing. Measurements should be made at the same time of day, ideally in the morning before breakfast and after the bladder has been emptied. For individuals able to stand, the most accurate type of scale to use is an upright beam scale that has movable weights. The individual should be weighed to the nearest 0.1 kg. For those that are not able to stand, a bed scale should be used. Tables are also available to estimate weight using recumbent measures.

Once an accurate weight is obtained, it should be evaluated by comparing the measured value to subjects of comparable age, height, and sex. To date, standards are not available for geriatric populations. Previously, weight comparison tables were available from the Metropolitan Life Insurance Company. These tables were developed using individuals of various heights and weights with the lowest mortality rates. The tables were developed using data for individuals up to age 59. As the aging process occurs, a higher percentage of body weight is adipose tissue, and body weight often increases as the percentage of lean body mass decreases.

The table developed in 1983 may be useful to use as a reference when weighing elderly patients. Determining frame size is also part of assessing weight status; however, there is no data available for determining appropriate frame size in elderly adults. The National Center for Health Statistics has reference data available from 1971-1974 in which height and weight measurements are available for individuals as old as 74 years of age.

**BMI**

Body mass index (BMI) is calculated dividing weight in kilograms by height in meters squared. BMI is used as an estimate of fat but does not take into account fat distribution or muscle mass. The Nutrition Screening Initiative (NSI) uses BMI to document nutritional risk in elderly adults; individuals with BMIs greater than 27 or less than 24 are at risk of poor nutritional status. BMI levels that are low may be correlated with a decline in functional status and an increase in mortality. One study showed individuals with a loss of one BMI unit per year resulted in a 35% greater chance of Alzheimer's disease than those who had no change in BMI. Conversely, women with higher postmenopausal BMIs had higher rates of breast and uterine cancer. Higher BMIs increase the risk of diabetes, heart disease and other chronic illnesses. BMI, however, was designed as an anthropometric tool when evaluating patients 25-65 years of age, and thus, accuracy and dependability may be variable when applied to older patients.

**Limitations of measurements**

Limitations of skinfold and circumference measurements in the older population are related to changes in body composition as a result of the normal aging process. Other factors that may affect the measurements are hydration, the elasticity of the skin and changes in subcutaneous fat. Also, because of the loss of fat stores in the extremities, the skin may be very loose on the arms, which may affect accuracy of measurements. Creatinine is formed by the metabolism of creatine and creatine phosphate that is found in muscle tissue. Creatinine height index uses the daily production of creatinine as a measure of total lean body mass. A limitation to using CHI in the older population is that it requires a 24-hour urine collection, which may be difficult to obtain. Also, there may be a reduction in creatinine excretion due to non-nutritional reasons as well as the presence of renal dysfunction, which affects urinary creatinine excretion.

**Nutrition-focused examination**

The purpose of a nutrition-focused physical examination is to identify possible nutrient deficiencies that may not otherwise be identified. A systems approach to the exam is used starting at the head and working downwards to the feet. The exam may be tailored for each individual using clinical judgment. Four techniques may be used to complete the exam and these may include inspection, palpation, percussion, and auscultation. Inspection involves using the senses to make observations about the condition of the individual's body including any potential nutrient deficiencies. Palpation involves using the hands to checking tenderness, size, pulsations, temperature, etc. Percussion involves tapping various parts of the body and interpreting the sounds in order to evaluate organs. Auscultation utilizes a stethoscope to listen to body sounds, such as bowel sounds or lung sounds. A nutrition-focused exam should focus on areas where deficiency signs are likely to be seen and may help to assess hydration status, presence of muscle or temporal wasting, skin condition and other signs of malnutrition.

## Adaptive equipment

An occupational therapist is an essential healthcare professional in assessing the need for and providing adaptive equipment used to facilitate eating and/or drinking. There are many adaptive devices available. Modified cups, such as those designed to aide in drinking and prevention of aspiration, are available to patients needing assistance. Spoons that have been modified to allow for placement of food in a specific area of the mouth are also available. Plate guards that fit over a regular dinner plate but allow the individual to more easily scoop the food onto their utensil are available. Additionally specialized mats that keep plates stationary are available. Mirrors are designed to assist individuals with facial weaknesses such that he/she may use the mirror to prevent food from pocketing in the cheeks.

## Malnutrition

Malnutrition is a common finding in the elderly population. Up to 50% of hospitalized elderly individuals and 40% of nursing home patients are malnourished. Clinical signs of malnutrition include weight loss, temporal wasting, loss of subcutaneous fat, and poor wound healing. Monitoring weight is one of the best ways to watch for malnutrition. Criteria useful in identifying malnutrition in nursing home residents include sadness (assessed on the Geriatric Depression Scale), cholesterol level less than 160 mg/dl, albumin less than 3.5 mg/dl, 5% or more weight loss and any type of eating disorder (physically or cognitively related). Malnutrition is associated with poor clinical outcome as well as increased mortality.

## Unplanned weight loss

In elderly patients, unplanned weight loss greater than 5%, over a 6-12 month period of time, requires a full evaluation. During the evaluation, a complete history should be obtained and the history of any symptoms relating to weight loss recorded. Diet, weight, social and psychological concerns should be noted. Additionally, risk factors leading to malnourishment should be discussed A complete physical exam, including an examination of the oral cavity, calculation of body mass index, assessment of subcutaneous fat loss and muscle wasting should also be obtained that. Moreover, laboratory assessments, including a complete blood count, serum albumin, cholesterol, liver function tests, thyroid stimulating hormone, electrolytes, calcium, glucose and renal function tests, ought to be performed. Stools may be checked for the presence of occult blood. X-rays may also be indicated. The cumulative results of these tests will help direct future care.

## Tube feedings initiation

There are many factors to take into consideration when deciding if tube feeding is an appropriate choice for an elderly patient. First, the individual's wishes must be taken into consideration. Available documentation such as a living will should be reviewed. The wishes of the individual should always take precedent over the wishes of family or caregiver if appropriate documentation is available to detail these wishes. The potential for improvement in overall quality of life must be considered. Any benefits to the individual's nutritional status must be weighed. Potential risks to the individual, such as the risk of aspiration, which may occur if tube feedings are poorly tolerated, must be considered. Tube feeding is not always the appropriate choice to make, and the overall plan for care should be evaluated. In other words, if other types of treatments are being withheld or withdrawn, the initiation of tube feedings needs to be weighed carefully.

# Nutrition Data Synthesis

**Assessing protein status**

<u>Serum albumin</u>

Measuring serum albumin level is one of the most effective and cost efficient methods available to assess protein status. Serum albumin is a visceral protein produced by the liver and has been shown to be a reliable prognostic indicator for hospitalized geriatric patients. Serum albumin is not greatly affected by aging although there may be a small decline in the rate of synthesis of albumin by the liver as an individual ages. Studies have shown that a serum albumin level less than 3.0 g/dl has been associated with increased mortality. One study, which examined Medicare patients, showed that low serum albumin levels coupled with weight loss positively correlated with higher rates of rehospitalization.

Caution needs to be taken in interpreting albumin levels as these may be affected by many factors. Dehydration may cause a false normal level while overhydration, such as that occurring with congestive heart failure, may cause levels to appear falsely low. In these cases, additional evaluation of protein status is required. Liver disease may also affect albumin synthesis thus causing a decline in serum levels. Albumin is also an acute phase reactant; therefore, the presence of any infection will adversely affect serum levels. Immobility may also cause lower albumin levels due to a decrease in nitrogen balance. When indicated, serum albumin may be used as a nutritional screening tool in elderly patients. Levels less than 3.5 g/dl may be indicative of protein calorie malnutrition and further investigation is warranted. Because of serum albumin's long half-life, tests will not likely show immediate response to nutrition intervention.

<u>Serum transferrin</u>

Serum transferrin is another major visceral protein. It is considered to be an accurate marker of protein status because the half-life of transferrin is only nine days compared to the three week half-life of serum albumin. There are, however, diagnostic limitations of serum transferring when applied to geriatric populations. As a person ages, tissue stores of iron increase, which in turn, causes a subsequent decrease in serum transferrin levels. This may cause false negative results in healthy patients and false positives in malnourished patients.

Retinol binding protein (RBP) is synthesized by the liver and is very sensitive to any factor affecting synthesis. RBP's half-life is only 12 hours, which makes it a very telling measure of malnutrition as well as a helpful tool for monitoring changes in nutritional status. Levels of RBP may be affected by liver or renal disease. RBP is also an acute phase reactant; thus, it is affected by infection or inflammation.

**Dietary assessment methods**

Nutritional assessment methods are tools used to identify individuals who are having difficulty eating an adequate diet, those who limit their food choices or exclude certain food groups, and/or those who follow an inappropriate diet. The aforementioned dietary issues may all lead to nutritional deficiencies. Assessment methods include 24-hour recall, diet history and food frequency logs, and food records. Obstacles to making proper assessment include skewed self-reporting due to memory loss or cognitive impairment; physical impairments impeding one's ability to read, write, or otherwise answer posed question; and visual impairments which affect one's ability to measure portion sizes. Often times, a caregiver, such as a spouse, child or close friend, assists with data gathering; however, this too presents obstacles.

<u>24-hour recall and food record</u>

A 24-hour recall is the most commonly used method for assessing food intake. An individual is asked to recall all food or liquid, and the amount of each, consumed within 24 hours. A better way to obtain this information for individuals in an institutional setting is by visual observation. A food record is also commonly used to assess dietary intake. A seven-day record is the most beneficial; however, many individuals are not motivated to complete this task for a whole week. A three-day food record is more manageable for most patients and is likely to be more accurate than a seven-day food record.

## A diet history with food frequency questionnaire

A diet history with food frequency questionnaire obtains generalized information on usual dietary patterns. Checklists may be used to simplify the process. Information that should be obtained includes food preferences, financial resources for obtaining food, ability to shop and prepare food and availability of cooking equipment. Information about special diets, alcohol consumption, and medication use should be obtained. Food preferences, to include ethnic and regional foods, should be noted. Both the quantity and type of food consumed should be obtained. The questions posed should be objective, include specific items, and portion sizes. Food models, photos and common household measures may be utilized to help obtain more accurate information. Simplified diet history and food frequency questionnaires are often used because the traditional assessment is often tedious.

## Fluid requirements

A general rule of thumb, for elderly population fluid requirements is that for every calorie consumed, one milliliter of fluid should also be consumed. An alternate recommendation is 30 ml of fluid for every kilogram of body weight. An elderly person typically requires between 1500 and 2000 ml of fluid per day. The ability to sense thirst decreases with age, and the mechanism that controls thirst is also affected, as the ability of the kidney to concentrate urine is reduced. Environmental factors that affect fluid intake are weather, humidity, and temperature. Changes in sweating may lead to altered fluid status. Endocrine factors that may affect fluid intake include changes in the renal angiotensin system. Physical factors, such as reduced mobility, may have an impact on one's hydration status. Chronic diseases also have an affect as may the presence of dysphagia. Additionally, one's fear of incontinence may adversely affect fluid intake. It is essential to impart the importance of having food and water readily available to clients and caretakers.

Dehydration

Signs of dehydration may include a quick, unexplained weight loss, and changes in the skin turgor or elasticity, especially seen on the skin of the back of the hand. Dry lips, mouth or tongue are also symptoms of dehydration. Dizziness and weakness are additional indicators of dehydration. As dehydration advances, a weak but quickened pulse, decline in body temperature, decrease in urine, concentrated urine, and/or confusion may be seen. Fainting, low blood pressure, convulsions and shock are possible if the dehydration is left untreated. Laboratory data may show elevated serum sodium, elevated blood urea nitrogen, elevated serum osmolality and elevated hematocrit. An elevated urine specific gravity may also be present.

Signs, causes of, and possible consequences of overhydration

Overhydration in a normal, healthy person is rarely caused by simply drinking too much water. Overhydration may be seen with congestive heart failure, liver disease, renal disease, Cushing's disease, or inappropriate antidiuretic or excessive fluid intake. The brain is the main organ affected by overhydration. Symptoms of overhydration may include depression, confusion, and drowsiness. Other symptoms may include blurred vision, changes in coordination, nausea, vomiting, and weakness. A sudden increase in weight may be seen. Laboratory data that may be noted include decreased serum sodium, decreased blood urea nitrogen, and decreased serum osmolality. A low urine specific gravity may also be seen.

## Assessing skin and nails

A nutrition-focused physical exam may show abnormalities in the skin such as poor wound healing that could be due to protein, vitamin C or zinc deficiency. It may also show dry, scaly skin or the presence of follicular hyperkeratosis that may be due to an essential fatty acid or vitamin A deficiency. Poor skin turgor may be observed that attributed to fluid intake. The presence of pellagrous dermatitis may be due to niacin deficiency. Easy bruising of multiple ecchymoses may be attributed to vitamin K deficiency. Fissures or cracks around the eyes or mouth may be indicative of niacin or riboflavin deficiency. Generalized pallor may be due to vitamin B12 or iron deficiency. Protein deficiency may also cause skin issues such as decubitus ulcers, dryness or dermatitis. Examination of the nails may show koilonychias (spoon-shaped) changes due to iron deficiency. Dull nails may indicate iron or protein deficiency, and pale, spotted nails may indicate vitamin A or C deficiency.

## Assessing oral abnormalities

A nutrition-focused physical exam may show abnormalities in various areas of the oral cavity. Cheilosis (fissures around the corners of the mouth) or redness of the lips may be attributed to riboflavin, niacin or pyridoxine deficiency. The tongue may be a site for presentation of B vitamin deficiencies. The color magenta on the tongue may indicate riboflavin deficiency. A tongue that appears smooth may indicate a deficiency of niacin, folate, riboflavin or B12. If the tongue appears red and swollen with changes noted in taste buds, one must consider deficiencies in niacin, riboflavin, folate, B12, or pyridoxine. A zinc deficiency may cause taste changes. Spongy and bleeding gums may be due to vitamin C deficiency. Iron

- 43 -

deficiency may also cause angular stomatitis and glossitis. An oral exam may also identify poor condition of teeth, the presence of a gag reflex, or improper alignment of the jaw, which may affect the ability to chew adequately.

Oral cavity

The three main functions of the oral cavity are chewing, initial digestion and speech. The chewing or mastication function is very important as this step prepares food for swallowing and digestion. The ability to adequately chew raw fruits and vegetables that contain the indigestible cellulose component is essential to proper digestion. Greater exposure to digestive enzymes increases the efficiency of the entire digestive process. Chewing also acts to stimulate the taste buds and contributes to the overall satisfaction of eating. The second function, initial digestion, begins in the mouth with saliva. Preliminary starch digestion occurs here with salivary amylase. The next step in this process is swallowing, which involves three stages: the voluntary stage, the pharyngeal stage, and the esophageal stage. The third function is speech. Speech involves a multitude of factors including respiration, resonation, articulation and oral sensation. Major influences of speech include the lips, tongue and soft palate.

Hard tissues in the oral cavity include bone, teeth, and the temporomandibular joint (TMJ). Age-related changes in bone include bone resorption and deposition. As the aging process occurs, bone resorption occurs at a lower rate, and over the age of forty, 1% bone mass may be lost per year. This is primarily seen in the alveolar bone and is a major contributor to periodontal disease and tooth loss. For individuals without teeth, alveolar bone loss affects the ability to comfortably and appropriately wear dentures. Teeth also experience age-related changes, such as changes to nerves and blood vessels. Moreover, the average life of human tooth pulp is estimated to be only 70 years. As aging occurs, tooth surfaces are flattened, and enamel is lost and is not reparable. This process contributes to greater tooth sensitivity and an overall higher pain threshold in elderly adults. The TMJ is involved in the chewing process, and it also undergoes changes throughout the aging process. Clicking of the joint, problems with the mandible and inability to fully open the jaw may be evidence that TMJ issues are occurring.

Soft tissues include the mucous membranes, periodontium, and the tongue. Atrophy of the oral mucous membranes is responsible for most of the changes affecting the epithelial layer. Signs that changes are occurring may include dryness of the mouth (xerostomia) and pain or burning anywhere within the oral cavity, especially on the tongue or palate. Environmental factors, such as smoking, may also contribute to atrophy of the membranes.

The periodontium includes the gingival and periodontal ligament. Gum tissue recedes with age and changes in health status, care of the oral cavity, and genetic factors may contribute to the progression of gum disease. The periodontal ligaments gradually loosen, which leads to root exposure and loosening of the teeth. Tongue changes also occur with age and/or may also be due to diseases or medications.

Dental disease
Universality refers to any disease of the oral cavity, such as dental caries or periodontal disease that may be seen throughout the age spectrum, not just in the elderly population. Irreversibility refers to diseases common to the oral cavity, such as tooth decay and bone loss, that cannot be repaired but may be treated to help prevent progression. Cumulativeness refers to structural changes in the teeth and alveolar bone that gradually occur over time. These three classifications of dental disease are not usually life threatening but may have a significant effect on an individual's social, psychological, financial and overall quality of life. Preventive dentistry is the single most important factor to preventing dental disease. Receiving regular dental checkups, at least annually, may prevent dental disease,

keep dental disease from recurring and prevent dental loss. Regular dental visits may also help to diagnose conditions and therefore, prompt early treatment. Individuals should receive regular dental care even if they are edentulous or wear dentures.

Oral cancer

Regular visits to the dentist may lead to early detection of oral cancer. Early signs may be white or red patches in the mouth, slightly raised lesions, or other subtle signs that may easily be detected by trained professionals. Other warning signs include oral ulcers, swelling, numbness or pain in the oral cavity, problems with swallowing, persistent unexplained bleeding, persistent sore throat and loose teeth. The most common type of oral cancer is squamous cell, which accounts for approximately 90% of oral cancer. Oral cancer occurs most often in older people, and age sixty is the average age for diagnosis. More men than women are diagnosed with oral cancer. The cause of oral cancer is still not clearly defined but the risk factors include the use of alcohol and tobacco products, poor diet, poor dentition, and sun exposure.

Xerostomia

Xerostomia is abnormally dry mouth. Xerostomia may be caused by medications, vitamin deficiencies, breathing through the mouth, and inadequate fluid intake. Certain systemic diseases, such as Alzheimer's, alcoholism, depression, diabetes mellitus, hypothyroid, lupus, nephritis, and rheumatoid arthritis, may cause xerostomia. Saliva acts to lubricate, cleanse and buffer the oral cavity and has antibacterial properties. With reduced amounts of saliva, there is an increased risk of developing dental caries, erosion of tooth surfaces, periodontal disease, and infection. Lack of saliva also affects speech and interferes with the adequacy of chewing and swallowing. Taste is also affected. Without adequate saliva, the ability to wear dentures is impaired. Mouth sores, pain along the gums, and generalized mouth pain while chewing is common. The range of consequences may range from mild to severe and may adversely affect nutritional intake.

## Assessing face, eyes, nose

A nutrition-focused physical exam may show abnormalities in face, eyes and nose. A moon shaped face or bilateral temporal wasting may indicate protein or calorie deficiencies. Generalized pallor in the face may be due to iron, folate or B12 deficiencies. If the eyes have pale conjunctiva, an iron, folate or B12 deficiency may be the cause. Vitamin A deficiency may cause multiple changes in the eyes. These changes may include night blindness, Bitot's spots, which are white, gray or yellow foamy spots on the whites of the eyes, corneas that appear milky white, keratomalacia or conjunctival xerosis, which is when the whites of the eyes appear dull or abnormally dry. If the nose has evidence of nasolabial seborrhea, which is yellowish, greasy material around the outside of the nose, a deficiency of riboflavin, niacin or pyridoxine should be assessed. If the individual is being considered for a nasogastric tube, the nose should be carefully examined for inflammation, presence of polyps or abnormal discharge.

## Assessing chest, lungs and heart

Any change in cardiac or pulmonary function should be fully evaluated by a qualified physician. Abnormalities in the chest/lung area may be identified upon a nutrition-focused examination. Protein-calorie deficiency may cause wasting of fat and somatic stores. Fast shallow breathing may be due to metabolic acidosis. Conversely, slow breathing, presence of apnea or cyanosis could indicate a metabolic alkalosis. Labored breathing may also be due to congestive heart failure. Non-nutritional reasons for changes in breathing may be due to multiple respiratory diseases such as chronic obstructive pulmonary disease (COPD). Some respiratory diseases may increase calorie expenditure because of an increase in the work of breathing. Irregular heart rhythms may be due to possible potassium deficiency. Fluid overload or deficit may be identified by the condition of the pulse. Heart palpitations could be due to hypoglycemic reaction. A thiamin deficiency may cause tachycardia and an enlarged heart.

## Assessing neurological abnormalities

Any change in neurological status should be fully evaluated by a qualified physician. General neuralgic function should be noted as this will affect overall nutritional status and ability to feed oneself. Hand to mouth coordination should be assessed. A deficiency of vitamin B6 may cause peripheral neuropathy or paresthesias, which is a tingling or prickly sensation on the skin for no apparent reason. Thiamin deficiency may cause confusion, irritability and weakness. Niacin deficiency may also cause confusion. A deficiency in folate or biotin may cause depression. Headaches, fatigue, apathy, and having problems sleeping may be due to pantothenic acid deficiency. Vitamin B12 deficiency may cause ataxia, an inability to coordinate muscle groups, paresthesias or mental disorders.

## Assessing musculo-skeletal abnormalities

Any change in musculo-skeletal status should be fully evaluated by a qualified physician. A nutrition-focused exam may identify problems with flexing, extending, or rotating the neck appropriately, which may adversely affect nutritional status by interfering with one's ability to self-feed. Muscle wasting on the arms or legs or saggy, folding skin on the buttock area may indicate protein-calorie malnutrition. Swollen and painful joints may be due to vitamin C deficiency. If the epiphyses or the end of the long bones are enlarged, a vitamin C or D deficiency should be evaluated. Vitamin D deficiency may also cause bowed legs, beading of the ribs (rachitic rosary) or other signs of rickets.

## Osteopenia

Osteopenia is a reduction in bone mass seen on x-ray. It is a form of metabolic bone disease, and the most common form is osteoporosis. Osteoporosis may be seen in the oral cavity. Alveolar bone loss is often the first sign of osteoporosis. This may lead to loss of bone in the mandible which may lead to tooth loss and/or the inability to comfortably wear dentures. Bone loss may also affect the shape of the jawbone and interfere with eating and speaking. Inadequate calcium intake, imbalances in calcium and phosphorus, smoking, caffeine, alcohol, certain medications such as steroids and lack of exercise also contribute to osteoporosis. Treatment may involve bone-building agents such as alendronate, vitamin D therapy, and exercise. Smoking cessation is also recommended as well as reducing alcohol and caffeine intake. The use of fluoride is also being explored.

## Sarcopenia

Sarcopenia is defined as loss of lean muscle associated with aging. The best way to evaluate how much muscle and adipose tissue has been lost is through skinfold and circumference measurements. Skinfold measurements are easy to determine and have been shown to correlate with body fat. The most common measurement sites are triceps, biceps, subscapular and suprailiac locations. The amount of fat and fat-free mass may be calculated using an equation that utilizes all four measurements. Circumference measurements may be taken from mid- arm muscle (MAC) or the calf. MAC measurements may be used with tricep skinfold to determine the arm-muscle circumference and the arm muscle area. Taken together these measurements may estimate how much muscle and lean tissue is in the body. Reference standards are available for comparison.

## Protein requirements

The recommended daily allowance of protein is 0.8 grams per kg for healthy adults of any age; however, some experts believe that protein requirements are closer to 1-1.2 grams per kg for elderly adults. Many geriatric patients do not consume adequate protein. Protein requirements are affected by changes in body fat and loss of muscle mass. The amount of exercise impacts protein requirements, as additional protein is needed to maintain protein stores. In fact, elderly adults who participate in high intensity exercise may require as many as 1.2-1.4 grams per kg. Other factors that affect protein requirements include liver and renal function as well as nutritional status. Testing serum albumin is a quick and relatively inexpensive way to assess protein stores. Serum albumin levels less than 2.1 g/dl may require additional protein in order to boost blood levels to normal ranges.

## Energy, carbohydrate and fat requirements

As a person ages, there is a concurrent decrease in metabolic rate coupled with changes in body composition. Often a decrease in physical activity and presence of chronic illness is often seen. Because of these factors, energy requirements are generally reduced in elderly populations.

Calorie requirements may be estimated a number of different ways. Generally, energy requirements for elderly patients may be calculated by applying 25-30 kcal per kilogram. Alternately, one may calculate the basal energy requirements and apply an activity factor to determine energy requirements. Carbohydrate requirements are estimated to be at 55-60% of total caloric intake. Increasing the amount of complex carbohydrates and fiber rich choices may help with bowel issues, diverticular disease, diabetes and hyperlipidemia. A goal of 25-35 grams of fiber per day is recommended. Fat intake should be limited to 30% or less of total calories, and only 8-10% of that from saturated fat. Controlling fat intake is an effective method of reducing calories and lowering the risk of obesity.

**Mucositis and stomatitis**

Mucositis is inflammation of the mucous membrane. Stomatitis is specifically inflammation of the mucous membranes in the mouth, including the lips, cheeks, tongue, gums, or palate. There are many causes of stomatitis including nutrient deficiencies, medications, breathing through the mouth, poor oral hygiene, allergic reactions or a burn from hot food or liquid. Many systemic diseases, such as inflammatory bowel disease, herpes viruses, leukemia, and HIV, may cause stomatitis. Radiation to the head and neck may also cause inflammation. The symptoms of stomatitis include pain or burning and difficulty swallowing. Stomatitis may lead to difficulty eating or drinking. Treatment involves relief of symptoms and removal of the inflammatory source. Topical anesthetics, such as lidocaine, may be used for short-term relief. Antacids may also provide relief. An oral paste, such as Orabase, may be used to protect the area. Avoidance of hard, sharp, and spicy foods is recommended.

**Side effects of medications**

Medications commonly prescribed to elderly adults may cause the following side effects (the list is not all inclusive):
- *Candidiasis:* Antibiotics, chemotherapy agents, corticosteroids, immunosuppressive agents
- *Excessive saliva production:* Anti-anxiety medications, lithium, nitrazepam
- *Mucositis:* Chemotherapy agents, lithium
- *Alterations in taste:* Benzodiazepines, chlorhexidine, levodopa, lincomycin, penicillin, propranolol, certain tranquilizers

- *Spontaneous bleeding in the mouth or intra-oral bleeding*: Anticoagulants, chemotherapy agents, aspirin and certain antibiotics
- *Xerostomia :* Amphetamines, anti-anxiety medications, antiarrhythmia, antidepressants, antidiarrheal, antihypertensives, anti-inflammatory, antipsychotics, benzodiazepines, decongestants, diuretics, lithium, MAO inhibitors, non-steroidal anti-inflammatory medications, tranquilizers
- *Excessive tooth decay:* Tricyclic antidepressants

## Dysphagia, aspiration and silent aspiration

*Dysphagia* is difficulty swallowing. Normal symptoms of dysphagia may include weight loss, an increase in secretions, changes in taste, or prolonged meal times, which may indicate the individual is taking longer to process the food bolus. A feeling of food stuck in the throat is a sign of dysphagia. Avoidance of certain foods, such as bread or meat, as these types of food are more difficult to swallow because they are drier and stickier, may also indicate dysphagia. Foods that do not form a moist bolus, such as rice or popcorn, may be avoided as well. An individual may add extra liquid to help swallow the bolus. These are all potential signs that an individual is experiencing dysphagia. *Aspiration* refers to the entrance of foreign material into the lungs during respiration. Coughing or choking when eating or drinking may signal aspiration. *Silent aspiration* is when aspiration occurs without symptoms such as coughing.

A speech language pathologist is a professional who is trained to assess, diagnose and treat disorders involving speech, communication, voice and swallowing. For an individual with dysphagia, the speech language pathologist may help the individual strengthen muscles involved in swallowing or teach strategies to compensate for impaired swallowing so the individual does not choke or aspirate. Tests available to diagnose dysphagia include a videofluoroscopic swallowing evaluation, fiberoptic endoscopy, ultrasound, MRI and CT scans.

Pneumonia is a classic sign of aspiration. Other signs of aspiration include coughing, a persistent low-grade fever, recurrent upper respiratory infections or recurrent pneumonia. Any change in lung sounds, an increase in secretions or a gurgle sound may be suggestive of aspiration and should be evaluated.

Phases of swallowing

Swallowing is largely a reflexive process. It begins consciously as one takes a bite of food but reflexes take over from there. The oral phase begins when food is taken into the mouth and chewing commences. Tongue action moves the food to the back of the mouth. Drooling and pocketing food may be indicative of an issue with the oral phase. Next, the pharyngeal phase is initiated. The nasopharynx closes to prevent regurgitation of food, and the airway becomes protected by the action of the larynx, the hyoid and vocal cords. The pharynx then contracts and allows the food to enter the esophagus. Coughing, gagging, and choking are evidence that there may be a problem in this phase. The esophageal phase is the final phase of swallowing. Once food enters the esophagus, movement is completely reflexive as the bolus enters the stomach. Mechanical obstruction or ineffective peristalsis will impact the esophageal phase of swallowing.

Conditions that may cause dysphagia

There are many causes of dysphagia. Neurological damage from a cerebrovascular accident or stroke is a primary cause. Parkinson's disease and neuromuscular diseases, such as amyotrophic lateral sclerosis, Guillain-Barre' Syndrome, or myasthenia gravis may cause dysphagia. Strictures, esophagitis, gastroesophageal reflux disease (GERD), and the presence of rings or webs in the esophagus may possibly impair swallow function. Different types of cancer, such as esophageal cancer, may cause swallowing difficulty as may surgery in the head and neck region. Certain medications may also impact swallow function. Individuals with altered and confused mental status are also at risk for dysphagia. Achalasia may impair swallow function because of weakening esophageal muscles. The normal aging process also increases the risk for dysphagia.

**The pancreas**

The pancreas has exocrine functions that assist with the digestion of fat, carbohydrates and protein, and endocrine functions that secrete insulin and glucagon. How aging directly affects the pancreas is still unclear but other factors such as nutritional status, liver disease, gastrointestinal surgery and medications may affect its function. Individuals over the age of seventy will likely experience some degree of pancreatic duct dilation. Typically 90% of secretion function must be lost before implications to the digestive process arise. Once 10% of pancreatic function is remaining, pancreatic insufficiency will be seen. This will ultimately affect fat, protein, and mineral digestion.

**Cardiovascular function**

The cardiovascular system is affected by aging and lifestyle choices, such as a decrease in physical activity. Continued and cumulative effects of poor dietary and lifestyle choices, genetic factors, and other unknown contributing factors influence overall cardiac function. Other age-related changes could include a gradual thickening of the vessels that leads to firmer, less flexible vessels. Arteries may also become dilated and the risk for aneurysm formation increases. These changes may also lead to atherosclerosis. The presence of hypertension and diabetes are additional contributors to the development of atherosclerosis. The types of lesions associated with atherosclerosis are fatty streaks, fibrous plaques and complicated lesions. Fatty streaks are strongly influenced by diet and may be reversible. Fibrous plaque and complicated lesions may lead to a gradual narrowing of the arteries and veins, which in turn leads to a decrease in blood flow. Ultimately these changes affect organ function.

## C-reactive protein and homocysteine

C-reactive protein (CRP) is an acute phase protein that is a marker of inflammation and has recently been used as a measure of heart disease risk. Elevated CRP has been linked to hypertension, obesity, and other risk factors. CRP should be measured in an individual who has multiple risk factors for heart disease. A level less than 1.0 mg/dl indicates low risk for developing cardiovascular disease. CRP levels between 1.0 – 2.0 mg/dl indicate average risk and levels greater than 3.0 mg/dl indicate high risk. Homocysteine is an amino acid found in the blood and elevated levels are linked to an elevated risk of developing heart disease, stroke or peripheral vascular disease. Elevated levels of homocysteine are thought to affect coagulation, promote the development of blood clots, and cause oxidative stress. Homocysteine levels are affected by genetics and diet, particularly consumption of folate, vitamin B6 and B12.

## Metabolic syndrome

Metabolic syndrome is a grouping of risk factors associated with the development of atherosclerosis and coronary heart disease (CHD). These risk factors include obesity (especially in cases were fat is primarily distributed across the abdomen), elevated fasting glucose levels, hyperlipidemia, and hypertension. Insulin resistance that leads to hyperinsulinemia is also a major factor to the onset of the metabolic syndrome. At least three risk factors must be present to diagnose the metabolic syndrome. The Adult Treatment Panel III (ATP III), as part of the National Cholesterol Education Program (NCEP), quantifies metabolic syndrome as three of the following: waist circumference greater than 102 cm in men and 88 cm in women; triglycerides greater than 150 mg/dl; HDL cholesterol less than 40 mg/dl in men and less than 50 mg/dl in women; systolic blood pressure greater than 130 mmHg and diastolic greater than 85 mmHg; and a fasting blood glucose greater than 110 mg/dl. Approximately 47 million people in the United States have the metabolic syndrome.

## LDL cholesterol

The main goal when initiating a cholesterol lowering plan is to improve LDL cholesterol levels in order to reduce overall cardiac risk. Elevated LDL cholesterol coupled with other risk factors has the most significant impact on cardiac risk. Factors that adversely affect LDL cholesterol are smoking, hypertension, low HDL cholesterol levels (less than 40 mg/dl), family history of heart disease (onset before age 55 in father or brother, 65 in mother or sister), and age greater than 45 years for men and 55 years for women. Initial treatment is geared towards lifestyle changes, such as lowering fat and cholesterol intake, increasing physical exercise and achieving a healthy weight.

## Obesity and CHD

The incidence of obesity is growing in the United States. Obesity is strongly correlated with the development of coronary heart disease (CHD) and is also strongly linked to high blood pressure and lipid levels (also risk factors for CHD). Many elderly adults do not get the recommended amount of daily physical activity, and as an individual ages, the quality of diet is likely to decrease. Distribution of fat also plays a significant role, with abdominal fat being the most dangerous and putting the individual at risk for developing the metabolic syndrome. The optimal BMI for adults is 25 but there is still no consensus on the optimal level for elderly adults. Studies have demonstrated that weight loss will reduce cardiac risk in elderly, overweight individuals.

## Regular physical exercise

Regular exercise is one way to help reduce many risk factors associated with coronary heart disease (CHD). These include blood pressure control, lipid reduction, blood glucose control and weight control. Exercise may also help relieve pain from osteoarthritis and osteoporosis by improving bone density and reducing hip and vertebral fractures. It also has positive effects on mental status, memory, mediating depression, and improving sleep quality. A healthy cardiovascular system helps an elderly individual maintain functional independence for a longer period. Exercise programs for elderly individuals may encompass aerobic activity, muscle strengthening, range of motion and flexibility exercises. Thirty minutes per day of moderate physical activity is recommended. This may be broken up into separate sessions if it makes achieving the goal easier. Any activity program should be started slowly and under the supervision of a medical doctor or other trained professional.

## Cholesterol lowering drugs

Three types of cholesterol lowering medication are as follows:
- *Statins:* These work by slowing the production of cholesterol by the liver and improve the liver's ability to remove cholesterol already present in the blood. Examples of statins include lovastatin, simvastatin, and pravastatin. Side effects may include upset stomach or cramps and muscle pain.
- *Bile acid sequestrants:* These are often used in conjunction with statins to lower LDL cholesterol by binding the cholesterol in the small intestine to allow excretion in the stool. Cholestyramine is one such bile acid sequestrant. Side effects may include nausea, constipation and gas.
- *Fibrates:* Fibrates work to lower triglyceride levels but are not effective at lowering LDL levels. Fibrates may increase HDL levels. Gemfibrozil is one

Copyright © Mometrix Media. You have been licensed one copy of this document for personal use only. Any other reproduction or redistribution is strictly prohibited. All rights reserved.

example of a fibrant. Gastrointestinal side effects are common and gallstone formation is possible.

Nicotinic acid and ezetimibe

*Nicotinic acid* is a form of niacin given in levels above usual recommendation to lower LDL and triglyceride levels and raise HDL levels. A common side effect is flushing of the skin as well as gastrointestinal symptoms such as nausea, vomiting, and diarrhea. The effect of high blood pressure medications may also be enhanced and should be watched closely. *Ezetimibe* may be used in conjunction with statins unless liver disease is a concern. Ezetimibe works to lower LDL cholesterol by blocking cholesterol absorption in the intestines. An example is Zetia. Side effects may include stomachache, muscle and joint pain, and allergic reactions in the face and throat area that may impede the ability to breathe.

Total cholesterol, HDL and LDL cholesterol and triglyceride levels

Total cholesterol, HDL and LDL cholesterol levels and triglycerides have all been shown to have a significant effect on the development of heart disease. Adults should have a lipid screen done every five years to monitor cholesterol and triglyceride levels. Abnormal levels will require follow up. Total cholesterol levels should be less than 200 mg/dl. LDL cholesterol, which is the type that causes the buildup of cholesterol in the arteries, should be less than 100 mg/dl. HDL cholesterol, which is the protective cholesterol, should greater than 40 mg/dl. Levels greater than 60 mg/dl are the most protective. Triglycerides, which are another type of blood lipid, should ideally be less than 150 mg/dl.

**The kidneys**

Age-related changes in kidney function begin around age forty. Generalized changes that may occur in renal function include a decrease in glomerular filtration rate, changes in renal perfusion, and decreased glucose resorption in the kidney. The kidney's ability to dilute and concentrate urine is also diminished. Urine may become more acidic due to the development of a chronic metabolic acidosis related, in part, to diet. The kidney also experiences changes in glomerular permeability leading to an increase in proteinuria. Additionally, the kidney gradually loses its ability to convert vitamin D to the active form (1,25-dihydroxyvitamin D). Older individuals with chronic conditions such as diabetes, hyperlipidemia, coronary artery disease, peripheral vascular disease and/or hypertension may experience a quicker decline in renal function than individuals without these chronic conditions.

Acute and chronic renal insufficiencies are commonly seen in elderly adults. Renal vascular disease, which may cause obstruction or acute renal failure, is possible. Renal failure due to nephrotoxicity from certain medications is more common in elderly adults. Proteinuria and hematuria may also be seen. The decrease in glomerular filtration rate and the decreased urine concentrating ability of the kidney in elderly adults may lead to the inability to effectively mange changes in fluid status. Also, there may be a build up of waste products from protein metabolism as well as electrolytes. This may lead to dietary modifications. Protein restriction is often recommended for elderly individuals with chronic kidney disease who are not receiving a form of dialysis. Generally 0.6 g protein per kilogram body weight is prescribed; however, one must carefully monitor protein intake to ensure daily needs are met and so as not to exasperate proteinuria. The recommended daily allowance for protein is 0.8 g/kg and amounts lower than this level may compromise nutritional status.

**Folate deficiency**

Folate deficiency causes megaloblastic, macrocytic anemia and may lead to generalized weakness, depression and neurological changes. Diagnosis is made by examining red blood cells and checking both a serum folate and a red blood cell folate. Serum folate levels do not necessarily reflect total body stores of folate. A vitamin B12 level should be checked as well to make sure this is not the cause of the megaloblastic anemia. Treatment regimen generally consists of 1 mg per day of oral folate. Folate deficiency is not common on its own but is usually caused by some other condition, such as chronic alcoholism coupled with deficient intake of folate or malabsorption. Medications such as phenytoin or trimethoprim may also cause a folate deficiency.

## B12 deficiency

Vitamin B12 deficiency is relatively common in elderly adults. The symptoms of which may include extreme fatigue, weakness, a red tongue and neurological symptoms such as dementia and numbness or tingling of the extremities. The heart is also affected by this deficiency because it has to work harder to pump blood. Pernicious anemia is the result of B12 deficiency and this is evidenced by a reduction in red blood cells. Vitamin B12 deficiency is usually caused by inadequate intake due to a meat-limited diet, as result of excessive alcohol intake, a lack of intrinsic factor in the stomach due to aging or surgery, or as a result of malabsorption, bacterial overgrowth, or H. pylori infection. The majority of individuals presenting with vitamin B12 deficiencies require repletion through intramuscular vitamin B12 injections.

## Iron deficiency anemia

Mortality risk increases in elderly adults with anemia. Iron deficiency anemia is common in hospitalized, elderly patients. The major cause of iron deficiency anemia is blood loss, often as a result of tumors or polyps in the gastrointestinal tract and/or cancer of the stomach or colon. Iron deficiency anemia may also result from genitourinary bleeding and/or cancer of the uterus or cervix. Blood loss due to peptic ulcer disease (either gastric or duodenal) may cause iron deficiency anemia. Hemorrhoids or diverticulitis may also contribute to the development of anemia. Multiple medications, including aspirin, non-steroidal anti-inflammatory medications and anticoagulants, may also be a causative factor of anemia. Screening for iron deficiency anemia should include a complete blood count and reticulocyte index and count. Serum ferritin and total iron binding capacity (TIBC) may also be helpful in diagnosing iron deficiency anemia. Generally, ferritin counts are low while TIBC levels are elevated.

**Pressure sores**

A pressure sore is a localized skin breakdown that occurs when there is continuous pressure or friction and a decrease in circulation to that area. Common sites for the development of pressure sores include heels, hips, buttocks, elbows, tailbone and coccyx. There are four stages of pressure sore development ranging from skin redness to deep openings extending to the bone or muscle. Risk factors for developing pressure sores include poor nutritional status, immobility, and infrequent position changes when bedridden. Other risk factors include diabetes, poor circulation, dementia, and incontinence. Smoking increases the risk.

Complications from pressure sores may develop and include infections that may be local or systemic, increased pain, and poor healing. Strategies to prevent pressure sores include frequent position changes and increasing mobility, minimizing rubbing or friction by using padding or pillows, the application and use of lubricants, proper skin care, the use of specialized mattresses, and proper nutrition.

## Bone mass

Peak bone mass occurs during the adolescent years, age 18 in girls and by around age 20 in boys. Sixty percent of bone mass is achieved during this period of rapid growth. Genetics has a major impact on bone mass, and lifestyle, physical activity, and adequate calcium intake also play large roles. Bone mass remains relatively stable until approximately age fifty. Initially, women lose bone mass quicker than men due to changes in estrogen levels. The start of menopause accelerates bone loss in women. Other factors that affect the rate of bone loss include changes in vitamin D metabolism, caused by less exposure to sunlight and a reduced ability of the skin and kidneys to convert vitamin D. Parathyroid hormone levels may also increase; this increase affects bone resorption and loss of bone mass.

## Elder abuse

Elder abuse is a very broad term. It may refer to physical, emotional or sexual abuse of an elderly person. It may also refer to neglecting to take care of an elderly person's physical, emotional or safety needs after agreeing to take responsibility for his/her care. The definition of elder abuse also encompasses intentionally harming an elderly and/or neglecting to provide care such that the neglect directly results in harm to the individual. Any type of exploitation of an elderly person, such as theft, fraud, control of finances or property is considered elder abuse. Most abusers are members of the individual's family and may be an adult child or spouse. Other abusers may be new acquaintances who target elderly victims. Abuse may occur at home or in a long-term care setting. Often times, the people who commit abuse against elderly adults have a history of drug or alcohol dependence, mental illness or personal stress.

Elder abuse is not always easily detected. An elderly individual may not be able to effectively communicate the abuse, or they may be afraid to disclose this information for fear of retribution. Warning signs of abuse may include burns or blisters, slap marks, or injuries that do not appear to be consistent with what is being reported by the elderly individual. Signs of emotional abuse may manifest as changes in normal behavior, mental status, or the appearance of new and unusual behaviors. Evidence of possible sexual abuse may include bruising or swelling around the genital area or breast or diagnosis of a sexually transmitted disease. Signs of neglect may include untreated pressure sores, absence of medical and dental care, issues with grooming, or unexplained weight loss. Signs of financial abuse may include changes in trusts or wills, suspicion loans to others, large bank withdrawals, or any unusual or unexpected change in financial situation.

## Elder self-neglect

Elder self-neglect refers to the inability of elderly adults to properly take care of their own needs or protect themselves from harm. Signs of self-neglect may include refusal to take medication or eat or the absence of readily accessible food. It may also include a lack of basic utilities such as electricity or heat. The inability to properly take care of grooming needs, such as bathing and manicuring fingernails, is a sign of self-neglect. Self-neglect may also present by the presence of accumulating trash or multiple animals living in the residence, both of which may lead an unclean and uninhabitable environment. Overlooking financial obligations may also indicate self-neglect Alcohol abuse or drug dependency may be a cause of self-neglect.

## Reporting requirements

In the case of suspected elder abuse, and if the individual is in immediate danger, the police should be contacted immediately. If the individual is not in immediate danger, local welfare or social service organizations will be able to help. Adult Protective Services (APS), which is part of individual state's human services division, is typically the agency that will investigate. After the report is made and deemed appropriate according to state law, the case is investigated. Otherwise, the case will be referred to an appropriate agency, where the case will be investigated, and the individual's safety is assessed. The caseworker will then develop a service plan that provides the necessary support, such as referral to an emergency shelter, legal services, or medical care. Victims of abuse do have the right to refuse services.

The passage of the Older Americans Act and formation of the Vulnerable Elder Rights Protection Program led the way for states to enact laws protecting elderly adults. The Vulnerable Elder Rights Protection Program helped to develop ombudsman offices and other support for elders. All 50 states and the District of Columbia have reporting laws although they vary greatly. Certain professional such as nurses, doctors, psychologists, social workers, and police are required to report abuse, but not all states require reporting of suspected abuse. There are currently no state laws that mandate that friends or family report suspected abuse of an elder. There is no formal federal funding for elder abuse programs, though some grant money is available. Each state administers Adult Protection Services (APS) independently and is financed mainly through state and local funds. Each state has an elder abuse hotline to report suspected abuse, and the phone call may be anonymous.

**Continuum of care**

The continuum of care is defined as coordinated care that involves diagnosis and treatment, and rehabilitative, supportive and maintenance services that address the needs of elderly adults. The needs address include health, social and personal needs. These services may take place in a variety of settings. Ambulatory settings include health centers, private physician offices, HMOs,

PPOs, and ambulatory care centers. Community based settings may include adult daycare, senior centers, and home health services. Institutional services may include hospitals, skilled nursing care and long term care facilities, rehabilitation facilities and hospices. Nutritional services that should be included within the scope of medical nutrition therapy include screening, assessment and ongoing monitoring and evaluation. Education, training and nutrition counseling should be included. Food assistance programs such as food stamps and meal assistance should be included. Case management and clinical care services are also extremely important.

## Malnutrition and respiratory function

Malnutrition and respiratory status are interrelated. Malnutrition may cause a loss of respiratory muscle mass (to include atrophy of the diaphragm) and may adversely affect overall lung function. Malnutrition also affects immune function and puts an individual at risk for infections. Malnutrition has been associated with increased mortality in individuals with chronic obstructive pulmonary disease. Low blood levels of nutrients, such as iron, calcium, magnesium or phosphorus, have a direct effect on lung function. Respiratory function is also adversely affected by protein deficiency in that the risk for developing pulmonary edema increases because of the decreased colloid oncotic pressure. Conversely, poor pulmonary function also impacts nutritional status. An individual with impaired respirations will expend more energy trying to breathe, which may lead to weight loss and loss of muscle mass. Calorie requirements are increased to account for this, however, it is often difficult to meet calorie requirements when it is difficult to breathe and eat at the same time.

Because many of the symptoms of HIV are commonly associated with aging, such as weight loss, fatigue or changes in mental status, geriatric patients infected with HIV are often diagnosed at a later stage in the illness, which makes treatment more difficult. . Furthermore, the stigma of being sexually active and having possibly contracted HIV may also prevent elderly adults from admitting symptoms in a timely manner.

## Dementia and tube feedings

Many individuals with dementia will develop problems with dysphagia over time. Placement of a percutaneous endoscopic gastrostomy (PEG) tube is becoming part of the standard of care for this population. This practice remains controversial. There are some studies that show improvement in functional status and increase in length of life with tube placement; however, other studies fail to show desirable outcomes, such as a longer life, less incidence of aspiration pneumonia, or improvement in healing of pressure sores, with tube placement. Many of the studies available are case studies and do not have control groups. Quality of life may be adversely affected by placement of a feeding tube, as restraints are frequently required to prevent the individual from dislodging the tube. Sometimes medication is used to reduce agitation caused by adding restraints. An alternative to tube feedings for dementia patients is hand feeding, which is time consuming and may not be a realistic option for individuals who do not receive one-on-one care.

# Nutrition Care Plan

**Specific care plan examples**

*An older man with difficulty chewing seeks advice on diet modifications to give foods a softer consistency.* Practical advice may help this man maintain a nutritious diet despite his difficulty swallowing. Additional fluids should be taken to try to assist with chewing and prevent dehydration. Attempting to maintain fiber intake is important and may be accomplished by adding bran to hot cereals and casseroles. Fresh fruits and vegetables may be prepared using liquids to soften the fiber, and mashing, chopping, and shredding fruits and vegetables may maintain some of the fiber. Protein sources that may be easier to swallow include fish, eggs, cheeses, yogurt, peanut butter, cooked beans and legumes, and ground meats. Trimming meats may also help remove some of the fibrous material that is difficult to chew. Adding meats and vegetables to soups or casseroles may help increase the nutrient content. A blender or food processor is a useful addition to the kitchen to make food softer. Cookbooks that provide recipes with softer consistencies are available to help this man prepare meals.

*The speech language pathologist has evaluated a patient for swallowing disorder. Compensatory strategies have been recommended including postural techniques and behavioral swallowing maneuvers.* Postural techniques are a way of repositioning or adjusting posture to aid swallowing function. Repositioning the head may prevent aspiration of liquids in as many as 80% of individuals with dysphagia. Examples of postural techniques include tucking the chin, which may improve airway protection, or turning the head to the affected side to direct bolus to the appropriate place. Behavioral swallowing maneuvers involve conscious strategies by the individual to help control swallowing. These may include consciously thinking about swallowing with each bite or swallowing more frequently. Other strategies may involve alternating liquids with solids. Many times strategies are paired to improve results. However, strategy use and/or results may be limited in populations with limited mental capacity.

## Environmental modifications

As an adult ages, changes in the swallow function will gradually evolve. This does not always indicate dysphagia; rather the elderly individual may be at risk for developing dysphagia based on age and other factors, such as medications or diseases. Sufficient time should always be allowed for an elderly individual to finish a meal. Eating or drinking while feeling rushed or hurried is not productive. Ideally, the meal time should be free from distractions, such as television, to allow the individual to concentrate on swallowing. If the individual has one side that is stronger than the other, the food should be chewed and swallowed on the stronger side. Adding fluids, sauces and gravies to increase moisture in a meal will facilitate the swallow function. Extra condiments such as jelly, butter or margarine, or mayonnaise may be added to moisten bread or crackers. Care should be taken to select items that fit within any dietary constraints.

## Texture modifications

Manipulating the consistency of food or liquid is a common recommendation to alleviate dysphagia. Thin liquids are often completely eliminated from the diet. Texture modification is difficult as there is no standard for texture/consistency modification. Often times, individuals are placed on a texture-modified diet but reevaluation is not completed in a timely manner; thus the quality of the diet may be impacted. Efforts have been made on a national level to standardize the language, consistency and interpretation of texture-modified diets. A task force called the National Dysphagia Diet Task Force (NDDTF) was formed and includes professionals from speech language pathology, dietetics, food science and the food industry. The goal is to have standard texture-modified diets that will enable healthcare professionals to choose the most appropriate diet.

**Thickening liquids**

There are multiple commercial products available for thickening liquids to a nectar, honey or pudding consistency. Powder and gel forms are available. Powdered products include but are not limited to: Thick-it, NutraThik, Thick & Easy, Thick & Clear and Thicken Up. Gel forms include Hydra-Aid and Simply Thick. Prethickened products including juices, coffee, water, milk and other drinks are available for purchase. Puree products are also available, including bread products and meals. These products are unique in that water is added and the product may be shaped to look like the actual product. It should be noted that many of these products are expensive, may not be covered by insurance and may be cost prohibitive to many individuals. Common food items that may also be used with appropriate guidance include banana flakes, cream of wheat, rice cereal, potato flakes, cornstarch, puree/baby foods, and unflavored gelatin powder.

The majority of commercial powdered thickeners use modified cornstarch and/or maltodextrin as the carbohydrate source. This contributes approximately 15 calories and approximately 5-10 mg of sodium per tablespoon. Most of the powdered products are gluten and lactose free and some are also kosher. Caution needs to be taken for individuals using powdered products as blood glucose levels may be affected. Because the powdered thickeners contribute calories to the diet, this may be an issue for individuals experiencing weight control issues. The commercial gel products use xanthan gum as the thickener and may also add preservatives such as citric acid or sodium benzoate. The gel thickeners contribute few calories because the carbohydrate is not digestible. The gel form also contains very little sodium.  Both products thicken fluids but once consumed, the fluid becomes available to the body for hydration purposes.

## DASH diet

DASH stands for Dietary Approaches to Stop Hypertension.  This was a trial that tested the effects of various foods on blood pressure.  The trial found that a diet heavy on fruits, vegetables, and lowfat dairy products and was low in fat, saturated fat and cholesterol had the greatest impact on blood pressure readings.  A second study was done called DASH-sodium that looked at reducing sodium intake.  This study showed the greatest benefits of the diet among patients who consumed less than 1500 mg per day of sodium.  The composition of the DASH diet is: 4-5 servings each of fruits and vegetables, 2-3 servings of non- or lowfat dairy, less than six ounces per day of lean protein source, 6-8 servings of whole grains, 4-5 servings per week of nuts or seeds, and 2-3 servings of fat per day.  Sweets are limited to less than five servings per week.

## Mediterranean diet

Research has shown that individuals over the age of seventy, who follow a Mediterranean diet coupled with a healthful lifestyle (exercise, non-smoking, etc.), may have a 50% lower mortality rate from diseases such as cancer, cardiovascular disease and coronary heart disease.  Additional research is suggesting that individuals with Alzheimer's disease who eat a Mediterranean diet may live longer than those who consume a traditional western diet.  The Mediterranean diet includes more vegetables and fruits than a traditional western diet.  It also involves a higher intake of monounsaturated fats such as olive oil or canola oil.  Intake of fish and poultry is preferred over red meat, and fish is consumed at least twice per week.  Nuts are included.  High fat dairy products are avoided and only low fat or fat free dairy are included.  With physician approval, an occasional glass of red wine may be consumed.

**National Dysphagia Diet**

Level 1: Dysphagia: Pureed

Pureed diet is indicated for individuals with moderate to severe dysphagia and with limited ability to protect their airway.  These individuals require close supervision while eating and often require alternative methods of nutrition support.  This is a puree diet that contains what is referred to as homogenous and cohesive foods by the National Dysphagia Diet Task Force (NDDTF).  This means the food has a pudding like consistency and does not contain any raw fruits or vegetables, nuts or other coarse foods.  The foods included do not require that a bolus be formed and do not need to be chewed or moved around the mouth in order for a swallow to occur.  Liquids may include thin liquids or those thickened to either a nectar, honey or pudding consistency.

Level 2:  Dysphagia: Mechanically Altered Characteristics

Mechanically Altered Characteristics is indicated for individuals who are able to make a transition from puree texture to semi-solid texture.  Individuals must be able to chew to some degree.  Individuals with mild to moderate dysphagia involving the oral or pharyngeal swallow are appropriate candidates for this level diet.  Individuals must form a bolus in the mouth, and the foods must have the ability to be cohesive.  The foods allowed for this level include all food from the previous level and any food that is moist and semi-solid.  Examples of foods included are ground meats, cooked cereals, pancakes, canned fruits, cooked soft vegetables, macaroni and cheese and other soft pastas.  Mixed texture foods such as soups and certain casseroles may require additional evaluation.  Liquids may include thin liquids or those thickened to either a nectar, honey or pudding consistency.

## Level 3: Dysphagia: Transition to Regular Diet

Transition to Regular Diet is indicated for individuals ready to make the transition to a regular diet. Individuals on this diet must have teeth or a well-fitting set of dentures and be able to chew well. Individuals with mild dysphagia involving the oral or pharyngeal phase should be able to tolerate this diet. Level 3 includes all foods from the prior two levels and regular texture foods. This level avoids crunchy, sticky and very hard to chew foods. Foods that have a moister consistency are preferred. Examples of foods that should be avoided include dry toast; crackers or cereals such as Shredded Wheat; any foods containing nuts or seeds; hard fresh fruits such as apples; fruits with difficult to chew skins such as grapes; vegetables such as lettuce, corn, and potato skins; tough, dry meats; and any chewy candy such as caramel or taffy candies. Liquids may include thin liquids or those thickened to either a nectar, honey or pudding consistency.

## Techniques to improve patient acceptance of the dysphagia diet

Individuals with dysphagia are often served unappealing, unappetizing foods just because the consistency of the diet needs to be modified. Because eating involves many of the senses including taste, smell and sight, attempts should be made to present food as attractively as possible. Seasoning pureed foods may provide a tempting aroma to stimulate appetite and increase the desire to eat. Layering pureed foods may help the appearance of the pureed item and may improve flavor as well. Pureed foods may also be piped onto a plate using a pastry bag rather than just placing on a plate without shape or interest. Pureed foods may also be molded to look like the food prior to the puree process. Garnishes are also important to adding interest, appeal and color to a plate. Taking the time to be creative and compassionate in providing meals for individuals with dysphagia helps these individuals maintain a sense of dignity and good nutritional status.

Nutrition support may be indicated for elderly adults with impaired swallow, especially in the early phases and until some function returns. The presence of dysphagia increases the risk for weight loss and malnutrition – both of which may compound the issues involving dysphagia. If an individual is at risk for aspiration, preventing pneumonia or sepsis is important. An alternative method of nutrition may be indicated if the individual is not able to resume an oral diet within seven days dysphagia onset and was well nourished prior to onset. If the gastrointestinal tract is functional, tube feedings are generally the recommended method of nutrition support. A nasogastric feeding tube may be used for short-term nutrition. For individuals requiring long-term support, a percutaneous endoscopic gastrostomy (PEG) may be placed. Tube feeding may also be used in conjunction with an oral diet. Often times, adding oral supplements and other calorie-dense foods will help maintain or improve nutritional status.

**Function of drugs**

The drug function and possible nutrient interactions are as follows:

- *Warfarin:* An anticoagulant. Vitamin K may affect metabolism. Intake of vitamin K should be kept consistent from day to day.
- *Cephalosporins:* A type of antibiotic that may cause vitamin K deficiency.
- *Isoniazid:* An agent used to treat tuberculosis and may cause deficiencies in vitamin B6 and niacin. It may also interfere with vitamin D metabolism and decrease calcium and phosphate absorption. Prophylactic vitamin B6 supplementation should be given at 25-50 mg per day and possibly a B-complex vitamin as well. Tyramine-containing foods should be avoided as this drug acts like an MAO inhibitor.
- *Metformin:* A type of biguanide oral hypoglycemia agent. This may decrease absorption of vitamin B12 and folate.

- *Alendronate:* A biphosphonate that may cause a decrease in serum calcium. A high calcium diet or calcium supplements should be taken. Alendronates need to be taken with plenty of water and on an empty stomach as absorption and effectiveness of the drug may be impaired otherwise.

- *Prednisone:* A corticosteroid that may decrease the absorption of calcium and may also increase urinary losses of calcium, potassium, zinc, and vitamin C. Calcium and vitamin D supplements should be taken to combat the risk for osteoporosis if long term use of prednisone is planned.

- *Digoxin:* A cardiac glycoside that may increase loss of magnesium in the urine and may decrease serum potassium levels. A diet rich in potassium and magnesium is recommended.

- *Hydralazine:* A peripheral vasodilator that may cause vitamin B6 deficiency. Supplementation with B6 may be indicated.

- *Cholestyramine:* A bile acid sequestrant that is also used to lower cholesterol. It may interfere with the absorption of the fat-soluble vitamins A, D, E, and K. The water soluble form of these vitamins should be supplemented or the usual form taken at least an hour before the medication is taken. It may also cause deficiencies of calcium, magnesium, iron, zinc and folate. The diet should be rich in these nutrients, or a supplement may be taken to prevent deficiencies.

- *Niacin:* A form of nicotinic acid sometimes used for cholesterol lowering. It may increase blood glucose levels and uric acid levels. Occasionally a low purine diet is needed.

- *Furosemide and bumetanide:* These drugs are loop diuretics that may increase urinary excretion of sodium, potassium, magnesium and calcium. Individuals undergoing these therapies should have electrolytes monitored and follow a diet rich in potassium, magnesium and calcium. A potassium supplement is sometimes required as well.

- *Hydrochlorothiazide:* A thiazide diuretic that increases urinary excretion of sodium, potassium, and magnesium, and may increase absorption of calcium in the kidneys. A diet rich in potassium and magnesium is recommended as well as close monitoring of electrolyte levels. Supplements may be required.

- *Spironolactone:* A potassium sparing diuretic that increases absorption of potassium in the kidneys. Potassium levels need to be monitored. The use of salt substitutes and potassium supplements are generally not required.

- *Acetaminophen:* An analgesic that may cause toxicity in the liver if consumed at high doses. The risk of liver toxicity is increased with chronic alcohol intake. Alcohol should be avoided while taking this drug or limited to less than two drinks per day.

- *NSAIDs:* Analgesics or anti-inflammatory agents that include ibuprofen and naproxen. This type of drug may cause gastrointestinal (GI) irritation and possibly bleeding. It should be taken with food or milk to help prevent GI effects.

- *Carbamazepine:* An anti-convulsant drug. It may cause deficiency of biotin, folate, and vitamin D. A diet that is high in B vitamins as well as vitamin D should be followed. As carbamazepine may cause bone loss, a vitamin D and calcium supplement may be needed for long-term use.

- *Phenytoin:* An anti-convulsant or anti-seizure drug. This drug may decrease serum levels of folate, biotin, thiamin, calcium and vitamin D. Long-term use may require supplementation of these nutrients. Phenytoin also interacts with enteral feeding and should be taken two hours before or after a feeding.

- *Phenobarbital:* A barbiturate based drug used to treat seizures. This drug may cause vitamin D and calcium deficiencies and may cause an increase in vitamin K metabolism. It may also reduce vitamin B12 and folate levels. Calcium, vitamin D, vitamin B12 and folate supplements may be needed for long-term use.

- *Lorazepam:* A benzodiazepine used to treat anxiety. Any benzodiazepine may cause extreme sedation. Alcohol should be avoided while taking this drug as it may further exacerbate the sedative effect. Caffeine should be limited as it will counteract effects of the drug.

- *Famotidine:* An H-2 blocker. H-2 blockers may reduce the absorption of vitamin B12 and iron, potentially leading to a deficiency. Iron studies and B12 levels should be monitored closely while taking this drug

- *Omeprazole and lansoprazole:* Proton pump inhibitors. Because less gastric acid is produced, absorption of vitamin B12 and iron may be affected. Supplementation may be added after weighing results of irons studies and B12 levels.

- *Metoclopramide:* A promotility agent that increases gastric emptying. Individuals with diabetes should be followed closely as this drug may affect blood glucose levels.

## Food and medication absorption

Medication use in elderly adults may affect food intake for many reasons. First, some medications may alter taste perception, which may already be impacted by the aging process. This may lead to disinterest in food because food is not as appealing. Next, certain medications may affect appetite level by causing anorexia or may conversely stimulate appetite. Also, medications may cause nutrient deficiencies that may lead to an alteration in food intake. Food may also affect drug absorption. This may occur as a result of a chemical or physical change. The ingestion of food may act as a barrier to absorption-site mucosal. Drug absorption may also be slower, enhanced or restricted due to the ingestion of food. Certain medications need to be taken on an empty stomach while others require food for optimal absorption. Close attention needs to be paid to the directions provided by the pharmacist.

## Hemoglobin A1c and blood glucose

The American Diabetes Association's recommendation for hemoglobin A1c levels falls at less than 7%. Other organizations, such as the Department of Veteran's Affairs and the American Geriatrics Society, take into consideration life expectancy, functional status and comorbidities. The recommendation for pre-meal blood glucose is 90-130 mg/dl. The peak after-meal blood glucose should be less than 180 mg/dl, and the blood glucose level at bedtime should be 110-150 mg/dl. A recent hospitalization may result in hypoglycemia because of an alteration in normal routine. Treatment with insulin or sulfonylurea medication may also contribute to hypoglycemia. Additionally, individuals experiencing cognitive illness may be at risk for hypoglycemia as they may not eat regularly. Individuals who have a complicated medical history, including diagnosis of diabetes mellitus or who take a multitude of medications are at risk for hypoglycemia. Beta blockers may hide the symptoms of hypoglycemia.

Classes of oral hypoglycemic agents

- *Sulfonylureas:* Agents used to stimulate the production of insulin in beta cells. This type of agent is contraindicated in individuals with sulfur allergies, liver dysfunction, and renal insufficiency. Examples of sulfonylureas include tolbutamide, glipizide, glyburide, and glimepiride.
- *Alpha-glucosidase inhibitors:* Agents work to slow digestion of complex carbohydrates and help maintain blood glucose levels after meals. Side effects include general gastrointestinal upset, bloating, nausea and gas. Contraindications include severe renal dysfunction and diseases of the small intestine. Examples of alpha-glucosidase inhibitors include acarbose and miglitol.

- 78 -

- *Thiazolidinediones:* Agents work to reduce insulin resistance and lower triglycerides while raising HDL levels. Side effects include fluid retention and leg swelling. Contraindications include congestive heart failure, liver and renal dysfunction, and edema. Examples of thiazolidinediones include pioglitazone or rosiglitazone.

Oral hypoglycemic agents

- *Meglitinides:* Agents work to stimulate beta cells to release insulin in response to elevated glucose levels. This type of agent may be better suited for those who have irregular eating habits; however, meglitinides have not been extensively studied in the geriatric population. Side effects may include nausea, vomiting, headache or joint pain. Contraindications include liver dysfunction, and certain drugs may increase or decrease the effectiveness of meglitinides. Examples of meglitinides include repaglinide and nateglinide.
- *Biguanides:* Agents lower liver glucose production. Side effects may include lactic acidosis, bloating, nausea, weight loss and vitamin B12 deficiency. Contraindications include renal and liver insufficiency and excessive alcohol intake. An individual older than eighty needs to have a normal creatinine clearance before this drug is prescribed. Examples of this type of agent are metformin and metformin/glyburide combination.

**Pharmacokinetics**

Pharmacokinetic refers to the interaction between a medication and the body regarding absorption, distribution, metabolism and excretion. Most medications are absorbed in the small intestine; therefore age-related changes to the gastrointestinal system would have an impact on absorption. This would include changes in gastric emptying and increases in gastric pH. It would also include decreases in gastrointestinal motility and secretions. Development of sarcopenia (loss of lean body mass) may lead to increased fat tissue, which may, in turn affect drug distribution. Decreases in cerebral blood flow and cardiac output also affect distribution. Age related changes in metabolism, such as liver dysfunction or changes in enzyme activity, play a major role in hepatic clearance of many medications. Finally, excretion of medication is affected by changes in kidney function, such as reduced glomerular function rate.

## Pharmacodynamics

Pharmacodynamic refers to the effect of drugs on the body. There are many age-related changes that may affect pharmacodynamics. These include changes in receptor sites or a reduction in the number of receptors. Changes in receptors are difficult to quantify because other factors, such as comorbidities or medications, may affect receptors. Homeostatic changes may also occur. In other words, as an individual ages, blood glucose levels, heart rate and blood pressure may become less manageable. Moreover, as an individual ages, he/she may become more susceptible to side effects of medications; thus tissue sensitivity may be a pharmacodynamic change. Additionally, changes in cardiac function may affect the heart's ability and response to medications. Changes in pancreatic function may affect medication-induced blood glucose response. Furthermore, changes in lung function may result in pronounced effects on respiratory function by drugs such as narcotic analgesics.

## Dietary supplements

Many elderly individuals use dietary supplements for a variety of reasons. It is important to note, however, that these supplements are often taken physician knowledge or supervision. One must use caution when adding supplements to a regimen as risks and effectiveness of such supplements are not entirely known. That being said, glucosamine and fish oil are commonly used to treat joint pain. Garlic is used for cholesterol control. Gingko biloba is often used to treat Alzheimer's disease and dementia. Gingko biloba is also thought to improve claudication in the legs. St. John's wart is commonly taken for depression. Kava is an herb used for anxiety. Valerian is used to treat sleep disorders. Saw palmetto is used by men to treat urinary problems, usually due to an enlarged prostrate.

**Megavitamin therapy**

Megavitamin therapy is defined as consuming greater than ten times the recommended dietary allowance of vitamins. Generally this is done because of a belief that it will help aid treatment of various diseases. There are negative implications to this practice. Too much vitamin E may interfere with warfarin and may cause a type of bleeding syndrome. Excessive amounts of vitamin D supplementation may cause hypercalcemia and cardiac arrhythmias. Excessive vitamin C may cause the urine to be more acidic and can lead to changes in how drugs are absorbed: acidic drugs will be absorbed easier while basic drugs will be excreted more rapidly if the urine is acidic. Vitamin C will also interfere with warfarin. Additionally, once high doses of vitamin C are stopped, a rebound effect resulting in scurvy is possible.

**Medications**

The most common types of prescription drugs used by geriatric populations are drugs used to treat cardiovascular illnesses. These drugs include diuretics, antiarrhythmics, antihypertensives, and anticoagulants. Psychopharmaceuticals are the next most commonly used category of drug and may include sedatives and neuroleptics. The third most common type of prescription drug used by geriatric populations is gastrointestinal drugs such as H2 blockers and laxatives.

The most common types of over-the-counter drugs taken by elderly individuals include analgesics such as acetaminophen or non-steroidal anti-inflammatory agents, antacids, antihistamines and vitamin supplements. *Polypharmacy* refers to prescribing multiple medications at the same time to treat the same disease. The major problem with polypharmacy practice is the confusion that results from keeping track of multiple drugs. Changes in mental status or functional status may complicate this issue. Polypharmacy may also lead to issues with medication compliance and increases the risk for drug-drug or drug-nutrient interactions. Medications prescribed for other conditions will also complicate the medication schedule.

Issues that affect medication compliance

In addition to the difficulties that arise from managing a complicated medication regimen, there are many other factors that may affect medication compliance in elderly populations. Issues with packaging may affect compliance if the individual is not able to open the container or dose the medication correctly, such as with insulin. Many elderly individuals do not understand how important it is to take a medication regularly and/or fail to take medicines as directed. Memory loss may also impact compliance in that an individual may skip a dose if they forget whether the dose has been taken; conversely, an elderly patient may accidentally overdose due to cognitive impairments. Confusion may arise if the pharmacist substitutes a generic drug, and the pill looks different. Financial concerns also play a significant role in compliance. Older adults on fixed or limited incomes may skip doses to stretch the prescription, take expired medications or share medicine with another individual.

## Alternative medicine

There are many different types of alternative medicine and therapies available. The use of herbal medicines is a growing trend. Massage therapy, acupuncture and chiropractic therapies are commonplace. Homeopathy, megavitamin therapy, and energy healing, such as magnetic therapies, are other types of alternative therapies. Common conditions that individuals treat with alternative therapies include chronic back pain, memory issues, headaches, anxiety, depression, sleep disorders, and arthritis. The Food and Drug Administration (FDA) does not regulate the herbal medicine market. Products may be sold without data that substantiates claims of treatment capabilities and safety. Additionally, product composition and dosing recommendations are not standardized. The FDA does not regulate the safety, purity, and quality control of herbs and caution should be taken in consuming any of these products.

## Drug-drug interaction

Drug-drug interaction refers to the interaction between different drugs (both prescription and over the counter) that may cause various side effects or may affect the action(s) of the drug(s), such as making the dose more potent. Some drug-drug interactions may be harmful. The risk for drug-drug interactions increases if more than one provider is prescribing medications or the individual has more than one condition for which medications are required. Conditions that increase the risk for drug-drug interactions include diabetes, cardiac arrhythmias, epilepsy, asthma or other respiratory diseases, liver disease, and thyroid conditions. The primary care physician and pharmacist should be aware of all medication an individual is taking including herbs, vitamin and mineral supplements, and over the counter medicine. Questions that should be asked include the chance of drug-drug or food-drug interactions, how the drug should be taken (i.e. with food or on an empty stomach), the drug's purpose, potential side effects to watch for, and signs of an interaction.

Warfarin has common drug interactions with the following drugs:

- Non-steroidal anti-inflammatory drugs (NSAIDs), such as ibuprofen and naproxen. The major interaction risk is severe gastrointestinal bleeding because NSAIDs may irritate and erode the lining of the stomach.
- Sulfa drugs, such as bactrim, may increase the effects of warfarin and the risk of bleeding.
- Macrolides, such as Zithromax or erythromycin, may also increase the risk for bleeding
- Quinolones, such as Cipro, Floxin or levoflaxin, also increase the effects of warfarin thus increasing the risk for bleeding.
- Phenytoin (Dilantin) may increase either the effect of warfarin or phenytoin. Prothrombin time, INR (international normalized ratio) and phenytoin levels should be monitored closely

ACE (angiotensin-converting enzyme) inhibitors, digoxin and theophylline have common drug interactions with the following drugs:

- ACE inhibitors and potassium supplements may interact to cause hyperkalemia because ACE inhibitors may decrease potassium excretion. Serum potassium needs to be monitored.
- ACE inhibitors and spironolactone may also cause hyperkalemia, and serum potassium should be closely monitored.
- Digoxin and amiodarone may interact with one another causing digoxin toxicity.
- Digoxin and verapamil may also cause digoxin toxicity and may lead to bradycardia or heart block.

- Theophylline and quinolones such as Cipro, levofloxacin or ofloxacin may cause theophylline toxicity because clearance of theophylline is hindered.

## Herb-drug interactions

Potential herb-drug interactions are as follows:

- Chondroitin sulfate may interact with aspirin or anticoagulants such as warfarin.
- Echinacea may interact with cyclosporine, which is used for immunosuppression, or with steroids, such as prednisone.
- Ephedra may interact with decongestants, caffeine, MAO inhibitors, digoxin, and other heart or blood pressure medications.
- Garlic may interact with aspirin, non-steroidal anti-inflammatory drugs (NSAIDs), anticoagulants, and certain diabetes medications.
- Gingko biloba may interact with aspirin, NSAIDs, anticoagulants, and diuretics.
- Glucosamine may interact with insulin or diuretics.
- Saw palmetto may interact with albuterol, anti-asthma medications and hormones.
- St. John's wort may interact with antidepressant medications such as sertraline or paroxetine, MAO inhibitors, theophylline, anticonvulsants, warfarin and many others.

## MNT covered Medicare Part B

In 2002, individuals with either diabetes or end stage kidney disease (not receiving dialysis) began receiving coverage for Medical Nutrition Therapy (MNT) under Medicare Part B. MNT is defined as nutritional diagnosis, nutrition therapy and counseling provided by a registered dietitian (RD). A physician referral is required to receive these services. RDs may now directly bill Medicare for services provided in regards to diabetes or renal disease. The American Dietetic Association developed a set of evidence-based nutrition practice guidelines/protocols for the delivery of MNT. These protocols detail the recommended number of visits required and what should be accomplished at each visit. Currently three hours of individual counseling are covered during the first year, and two hours are covered in each subsequent year. Additional visits may be extended based on physician input. At this time, there is no direct MNT Medicare coverage for conditions or diseases such as obesity or hyperlipidemia.

**Medicare reimbursement conditions**

Medicare reimbursement to hospitals and skilled nursing facilities are based on diagnosis-related groups (DRGs). Each DRG is reimbursed at a flat rate, and the number of services a patient receives is not taken into account, just the individual DRG. In order to be eligible for Medicare reimbursement, there are multiple conditions that need to be met. Nutrition related services requirements include the presence of an organized nutrition department that provides food service and nutritional care. At minimum, a consulting dietitian needs to be available to provide nutrition assessment, obtain diet histories, provide education regarding therapeutic diets, provide in-services to physician and nursing staff, and be available for patient care conferences. Written orders for modified and therapeutic diets must be obtained and included in the patient's medical record. Additionally, meals served to patients must comply with all diet restrictions.

Nutrition services for conditions other than diabetes or end-stage kidney disease may be covered under Medicare Part B if the service is considered "incident to medical care." This means the service must be part of care already being provided at the time the patient is seen. Generally, the registered dietician (RD) must be an employee of the physician practice or hospital in order for the services to be billed to Medicare. Most RDs act as consultants and are not employees of the physician practices for whom they consult. This creates a barrier for reimbursement for important nutrition services. An HMO that participates in the Medicare program typically provides the same level of service for all its patients, and some nutrition services are reimbursed.

**USDA dietary guidelines**

The USDA dietary guidelines were originally released in 1980 and updated in 2005. The main goal of these guidelines was to provide advice on the positive impact that a healthful diet may have on prevention of chronic disease. Key recommendations include consuming a variety of foods and drinks while limiting intake of total, saturated and trans fats. The guidelines advise individuals to maintain ideal weights. Moreover, the guidelines encourage regular physical activity. The guidelines also include recommendations, such as consuming at least four cups combined of fruits and vegetables, eating whole grain products and low fat dairy products. Increasing fiber intake is recommended as well. A sodium limit of 2300 mg per day is suggested, and the consumption of potassium rich foods is advised. Alcohol intake should be limited to one drink per day for women and two for men. Finally, the guidelines address food safety issues.

**Food Guide Pyramid**

The Food Guide Pyramid replaced the basic four food groups in 1990. The premise is based on a pyramid shape with the base of the pyramid indicating healthier foods and the top of the pyramid indicating less healthy foods, which should be eaten sparingly. The Food Guide Pyramid was developed in part to assist individuals with making appropriate food selections as recommended by the USDA Dietary Guidelines. The Food Guide Pyramid recommends 6-11 servings of whole grains per day, 2-4 servings of fruit, 3-5 servings of vegetables, 2-3 servings of meat or meat substitute, and 2-3 servings of dairy products. It is a general guide and provides appropriate serving sizes. Researchers from Tufts University are lobbying for adoption of an over-70 pyramid that stresses adequate hydration, calorie reduction to prevent weight gain, and supplements of calcium, vitamin D and B12 to prevent deficiencies among geriatric populations.

## RDAs and DRIs

RDAs were originally established in 1941 as general guidelines for nutrient intake and to prevent deficiencies. They were developed for healthy people. In contrast, the DRIs were developed as estimates of appropriate nutrient intakes for healthy individuals. DRIs aid in planning nutritionally complete diets. DRIs include tolerable upper limits (TUL), which quantify the largest intake of a nutrient such that it will not result in adverse effects in healthy individuals. DRIs also include estimated average requirements (EAR), which are the nutrient intake values estimated to be safe for 50% of the population. Adequate intake (AI) is the benchmark intake for nutrients without an RDA established. The RDA is also included in DRIs and refers to average intake of a nutrient that will prevent deficiency in 98% of the population. In general, for elderly patients, RDA or AI will be higher for vitamin D but the recommendations for other nutrients remain fairly consistent.

## NCI and ACS

The general recommendations from the National Cancer Institute (NCI) and the American Cancer Society (ACS) to reduce cancer risk are to choose more plant-based foods and eat at least five servings per day of fruits and vegetables. Soy products and legumes are encouraged. Whole grains should be selected more often than more refined carbohydrates. Fat intake should be limited. Red meat should be restricted. Foods should be baked or broiled rather than fried. Physical activity should be increased to at least 30 minutes per day and a healthy weight should be achieved and maintained. Alcohol intake should be limited to two drinks per day or less, and smoking should be avoided.

## General housing options

There are a number of housing options available for elderly individuals of all abilities. For independent living, there are senior apartments that allow for self care but have adaptive equipment installed for assistance. Senior housing is also available to lower income elderly adults. Additionally, there are housing options that provide a variety of services. These include assisted living, which provides assistance with personal care, meals and housekeeping. Board and care is also a frequently offered housing option, and this option generally includes a smaller living space, such as a room, along with meals and personal care. Continuing care retirement communities provide living accommodations that offer a full range of options from independent living to assisted living to nursing home care all within the same community. Finally, there is the nursing home option for individuals who can no longer care for themselves. This may be short term, long term or for rehabilitative purposes.

## Adult daycare programs

There are typically three types of adult day care programs: social, health and a combination social/health. The social programs are geared towards seniors who are high functioning and require minimal assistance. Meals are provided and special diets may be accommodated. Activities are planned to include all seniors, and many programs include music, arts and crafts, games, low-level exercise, and discussion groups. Field trips to places of interest are often planned as well. The adult day health programs and combination programs have a staff nurse who is available to provide medications and may also provide tracheotomy care and tube feedings. Nursing assistants are also on staff to assist with personal care needs. The benefits of these types of programs include social stimulation, nutritional meals, safe environments, improved mental and physical well-being, and improved levels of independence.

**Discharge planning**

Discharge planning is a process that determines the care required to ensure a patient's needs are met as the patient is transferred from one level or type of care to another. This is an important process because as hospital lengths of stay shorten, many patients require some sort of additional care after discharge. Discharge planning could include transfer to a skilled nursing facility, nursing home or rehabilitation hospital. It could also include transfer to the individual's home with the provision of home care services such as nursing care. Any hospital that accepts Medicare payments must legally provide a detailed, written discharge plan to the patient. The hospital personnel responsible for the discharge plan may be an RN, social worker, or case manager/utilization reviewer. The discharge plan should be interdisciplinary as well.

There are three basic components to a discharge plan: planning, training, and referrals. Planning for discharge starts upon admission to the hospital. Planning involves determining what services Medicare will cover for the patient and what services the patient may be responsible for paying. It will also include determining what services will be needed at homed or the type of facility the patient may need at discharge. Transportation need must be arranged. For any home care, all supplies, equipment and modifications to the home need to be arranged. Follow-up appointments should also be scheduled.

The training process of a discharge plan should involve medication instruction, including type of drug, dose, function and possible side effects. It also involves teaching the patient or caregiver skills needed to function at home, including equipment instruction, special procedures involved in care, or disease management.

The final process of the discharge plan is the referral process. It involves making referrals to community agencies that offer needed services, such as equipment, home care services (i.e., home health aide), transportation services, and others.

## Xerostomia

Management of xerostomia is directed at alleviating symptoms. If xerostomia is due to medication use, substituting another medication or reducing the dosage or frequency of the medication should be considered. Increased fluid intake and the use of humidified air is often helpful. Alcohol and tobacco should be avoided. The use of artificial saliva may be useful, and this works by providing lubrication to the mucosa. Lidocaine, pilocarpine drops, and glycerin swaps are sometimes prescribed to help manage pain. Consuming sugarless candy or gum may also alleviate symptoms; however, care must be taken to avoid over consumption of this type of product as they may adversely affect gastrointestinal function if sorbitol is a main ingredient. Lemon flavored candies and gums are not recommended as they may cause a drying effect. Vaseline or petroleum jelly may also relieve symptoms. Because there is an increase in the risk for developing dental diseases, frequent dental evaluations are recommended. Diet modifications such as modifying texture of food are helpful as well.

**Strokes**

A stroke is also called a cerebrovascular accident (CVA) and occurs when there is an interruption of blood to the brain. An ischemic type is the most common form of stroke, and this occurs when a blood clot blocks the flow of blood to the brain. This is most commonly seen in individuals with atherosclerosis. The risk factors for stroke include family history, age, smoking, hypertension, diabetes, elevated lipids, obesity and excessive weight gain. Preventive measures include eating a healthy diet that is low in fat and high in fresh fruits and vegetables. Regular blood pressure screening as well as cholesterol screening is important. Total cholesterol should be less than 200 mg/dl and LDL cholesterol should be less than 70 mg/dl. The use of cholesterol lowering medications may be necessary. Smoking cessation, limiting alcohol intake and regular, aerobic exercise are also preventive measures that may be taken

**Gastritis and gastric acid**

Gastric acid secretion may be caused by many factors including certain medications, such as aspirin and steroids, non-steroidal anti-inflammatory drugs (NSAID), alcohol, chronic vomiting, infections, and autoimmune factors involving the stomach. It may also be caused by *Helicobacter pylori* infection. This can lead to chronic inflammatory gastritis, which in turn, may cause atrophic gastritis. Atrophic gastritis may cause a loss of gastric glands that will make healing of the gastric epithelium unlikely. The consequences of chronic gastritis and reduced acid secretion include the development of vitamin B12 deficiency or pernicious anemia. It may also lead to bacterial overgrowth syndrome because of the protective effect that gastric acid has on the growth of bacteria in the gut. The risk of developing a gastric ulcer also increases.

Because antacids are sometimes used to treat gastritis and gastric ulcers, elderly adults are at risk for experiencing side effects of antacid therapy.

**Celiac disease**

Celiac disease has historically been associated with younger people. With improved detection tests, new cases are being seen among populations in their forties and seventies. As many as 33% of new cases present in individuals over the age of sixty. The clinical presentation of celiac disease in elderly adults is different from that of younger people. Only about 25% of elderly adults present with diarrhea or weight loss. The main symptoms tend to be gastrointestinal distress and suboptimal health. Many elderly individuals who present with celiac disease may have a number of vitamin and mineral deficiencies including folate, iron, vitamin D and calcium deficiencies. Osteopenia or osteoporosis may be present as well.

During diagnosis of celiac disease, specific antibodies may be identified. A small bowel biopsy may diagnose celiac disease. Treatment involves the implementation of a gluten free diet and close assistance of a registered dietician (RD). The RD will aid patient dietary modifications and adaptations. Vitamin and mineral repletion is also required.

**Congestive heart failure (CHF)**

Congestive heart failure is a condition that occurs as a result of left ventricular dysfunction that causes edema, fatigue and shortness of breath. This occurs as a result of the heart being unable to properly circulate blood throughout the body. The incidence of CHF increases with age but at around age 75, the incidence increases substantially. This increased risk is most likely due to age-related changes in cardiac function coupled with other factors, such as hypertension or valve disease. Primary CHF treatment involves the use of diuretics, exercise, and diet. A low sodium diet is indicated and an intake of 3000 mg per day or less is ideal. For individuals with moderate or severe disease, a further sodium reduction to less than 2000 mg per day may be required. Fluid restriction is often required as well.

Energy requirements

Energy requirements for individuals with CHF are dependent upon the individual's current height and weight, level of activity and degree of CHF. For overweight or obese individuals who are not able to increase their activity level, calorie intake must be reduced in order to attempt a more appropriate body weight. For malnourished individuals with CHF, calorie requirements may be increased up to 50% above basal requirements to compensate for increased energy expenditure caused by respiratory distress. Many CHF patients require 35 kcal/kg to meet energy requirements.

Cardiac cachexia

Cardiac cachexia is a type of starvation seen in up to 50% of individuals with moderate to severe CHF. Depletion of fat and protein stores is evident and immune function is poor. There is also a significant loss of lean body mass, which includes loss of cardiac muscle. Small, frequent meals and snacks are recommended as eating full meals often require more energy. Moreover, larger meals cause a full abdomen which impacts breathing and increases oxygen consumption. The use of high calorie supplements is beneficial.

**Cardiovascular disease (CVD)**

Cardiovascular disease (CVD) is the leading cause of death in the United States. As many as 40% of adults over the age of 65 have some form of heart disease. As an individual ages, the risk increases. It is estimated that by age 65, at least 50% of individuals will experience a significant cardiac event. Often times, symptoms in an elderly individual may not be recognized because of advancing age. Symptoms may present as reduced ability to engage in physical activity, though this may be attributed to aging. There are multiple risk factors for developing heart disease. Some are preventable while others, such as male gender and family history, are not. Measures that may be taken to reduce risk include smoking cessation, increasing exercise, achieving and maintaining a healthy body weight, controlling hypertension and diabetes, and controlling blood lipid levels through diet and/or medication.

## COPD

COPD is a type of pulmonary disease characterized by obstructed airflow, usually caused by emphysema or bronchitis. The use of bronchodilators may alleviate symptoms, but the condition is usually irreversible. An individual with COPD should receive a full nutrition assessment. Reduced food intake is a common change related to decrease respiratory health. Becoming tired easily or having difficulty chewing and swallowing are also common. Changes in gastrointestinal function are also possible, especially if a low fiber diet is consumed. Calorie requirements should be evaluated as energy requirements are sometimes elevated. However, some individuals with COPD should lose weight. Adequate calorie consumption is important in order to spare protein stores. Protein requirements are usually 1.2-1.7 grams per kg of dry weight, and nutrient intake should be balanced with 30-45% of calories from fat and approximately 40-55% of calories from carbohydrates. Meeting the dietary reference intakes (DRIs) for vitamins and minerals is important.

An oral diet modified for texture is usually indicated for patients with COPD. Additionally, a fiber source should be included to manage bowel health. The use of oxygen during meal times is often required to increase endurance while attempting to eat. Other dietary suggestions include chewing foods slowly and thoroughly, maintaining proper position while eating and paying attention to swallowing to prevent aspiration. Assistance with shopping and meal preparation is important. Participation in nutritional programs for elderly adults, such as Meals on Wheels, or congregate meals should be considered. Nutritional supplementation with high calorie drinks is often recommended as a way to increase caloric intake. Occasionally, tube feeding is indicated in order to improve nutritional status and quality of life. This may be provided nocturnally to supplement caloric intake during the day.

**Wound healing**

Adequate nutrition is essential to wound healing. Energy requirements should be estimated based on individualized weight, activity level, comorbid diseases, stage and size of the pressure sore, stage of healing process and overall nutritional status. Calorie requirements may be as high as 30-35 kcal/kg. Underweight individuals, patients experiencing continued weight loss, or requiring additional calories to stimulate wound healing may require as much as 40 kcal/kg daily. Adequate protein intake is extremely important as it plays a role in collagen formation and overall skin integrity. Protein requirements are estimated at 1.25-1.5 grams per kg per day for healing. Adequate hydration is also important for healing. Specific vitamins associated with wound healing include vitamins A, C, E, and zinc. Iron and vitamin K are also important.

**Parkinson's disease**

Parkinson's disease (PD) is a neurological disorder associated with a decrease in dopamine production and is characterized by rigidity of muscles, tremors at rest, a shuffling gait, and difficulty with balance. Over 60% of those diagnosed with PD will become disabled within five years. Medical nutrition therapy involves consuming regular meals and snacks and meeting the daily reference intakes for nutrients. Individuals with PD are at risk for developing osteoporosis. Maintaining appropriate intake of calcium and vitamin D is essential for good bone health. Constipation is a common issue with PD. Consuming adequate amounts of fiber and fluids is important to help regulate bowels and prevent obstruction. Dietary protein may interfere with the use of levodopa containing medications such as Sinemet, causing the drug to be less effective. Portions of meat should be limited to the size of a deck of cards, and the levodopa containing medication should be taken at least thirty minutes prior to eating.

## Osteoarthritis

Osteoarthritis (OA) is the most common form of arthritis in elderly adults. OA is a degenerative disease that occurs when the cartilage wears away leaving the bones to rub against each other. This causes pain and stiffness in the joints. Aging, being overweight, and having injuries to joints are risk factors for developing OA. Achieving and maintaining a healthy weight is imperative for effective treatment of OA. A well balanced diet is recommended. Herbs and supplements are often used to treat symptoms of OA. This should be done with caution and under a physician's supervision. According to the Arthritis Foundation, two supplements that may be helpful are glucosamine and chondroitin. The use of these supplements should be discussed with the treating physician.

## Unplanned weight loss

The first step in treating weight loss is to assess calorie and protein requirements. Many elderly adults will require approximately 30-35 kcal/kg daily to regain weight. Protein requirements may vary from 1-1.5 g/kg daily depending upon protein status. A well balanced diet with a multivitamin supplement is recommended. The use of nutrition programs for elderly adults should be investigated. Small frequent meals are often helpful to maximize intake. Nutritional supplements may be utilized as an extra calorie source and may be especially beneficial if provided between meals. Assistance during meals is recommended. Exercise, if medically appropriate, may be a good way to stimulate appetite. There are also pharmacological approaches that may be used but not as the first choice of treatment. The use of appetite stimulants has not been extensively studied in the geriatric population but choices of stimulants include Megestrol, tetrahydrocannabinol, and oxandrolone. Outcomes that may be expected include weight gain or weight maintenance, improved quality of life, increased serum albumin levels, and improvement in functional status.

## Hypertension

Over 65 million adults have high blood pressure and more than 50% of all adults over the age of sixty have hypertension. These individuals have a higher risk of dying from a stroke, heart disease or kidney failure. African Americans are at higher risk for developing hypertension. Hypertension is more prevalent in males over the age of 45 and in females over the age of 55. Additional risk factors being overweight or obese, a positive family history of hypertension, excessive salt intake, alcohol consumption, smoking, stress, lack of exercise, and inadequate potassium in the diet. Certain medications such as steroids, decongestants, and antidepressants may also elevate blood pressure.

Hypertension is common among elderly adults and the definition does not vary between age groups. Healthy blood pressure is less than 120 mmHg/80 mmHg. Prehypertension is defined as a systolic blood pressure reading between 120-139 mmHg and a diastolic reading of 80-89 mmHg. Stage 1 hypertension is diagnosed when blood pressure falls between 140-159 mmHg/90-99 mmHg. Stage 2 hypertension is classified as a systolic reading greater than 160 mmHg and a diastolic reading over 100mmHg. Hypertension is often referred to as the silent killer because the symptoms are not obvious. Untreated hypertension is very dangerous and may affect arteries and may lead to heart and kidney disease. Hypertension may also affect the eyes and brain, ultimately leading to a stroke.

<u>Preventing hypertension</u>

Prevention of high blood pressure is possible. Some steps that may be taken to help with this include:

- Achieving and maintaining a healthy weight. Even a loss of 10 pounds may greatly influence blood pressure.
- Reducing salt and sodium intake to less than 2400 mg per day.
- Improving overall eating habits to more healthful choices. The DASH diet is often recommended.
- Increasing physical activity is important. A goal of at least 30 minutes of moderate exercise, such as walking, yard work and gardening, and even wheeling oneself in a wheel chair if physically impaired is recommended.
- Limiting alcohol intake to less than one drink per day for women and less than two for men.
- Smoking cessation.


<u>Drug therapy for hypertension</u>

Older individuals may benefit from controlled blood pressure just as much as younger adults. Any individual who has abnormal blood pressure readings should begin to implement lifestyle changes to help improve blood pressure. Drug therapy is usually started for individuals who have stage one or two hypertension. Thiazide diuretics are generally the first medication prescribed to treat hypertension. These help the body get rid of excess fluid and sodium by excretion through the kidney. Other types of blood pressure medications include beta-blockers, calcium channel blockers, angiotensin converting enzyme (ACE) inhibitors, angiotensin antagonists, alpha-blockers and vasodilators. Often times, different types of blood pressure medications are prescribed at the same time to optimize treatment.

## Diabetes Mellitus

In elderly patients, diabetes often presents with vague, non-specific symptoms such as fatigue, dizziness, increasing frequency of falls, and confusion. Often DM may present as a urinary tract infection or an individual may experience excessive urination, especially at night. Weight loss may also be a symptom. The classic symptoms of DM in elderly adults may not occur until serum glucose levels are greater than 200 mg/dl. These symptoms may include blurred vision, hunger, thirst and excessive urination. The American Diabetes Association recommends that screening for diabetes begin at age 45. At that time and every three subsequent years, a fasting glucose check ought to be performed. These screening guidelines may not be adequate, however, given the rising incidence of diabetes and the increased elderly population who have multiple risk factors for the development of DM.

Prevalence

As many as 40% of adults over the age of 75 have either glucose intolerance or diabetes mellitus (DM). Additionally, the incidence of individuals with metabolic syndrome (insulin resistance, elevated lipids, high blood pressure and obesity) is greatest among individuals aged 65 to 75 than it is in any other age group. The incidence is increasing and certain groups, such as Native Americans, Hispanics, and African Americans, are at greater risk for developing diabetes. Factors that contribute to the development of DM include age-related reduction in pancreatic beta cell function as well as reduced insulin production and insulin resistance. Obesity, limited physical activity and changes in body composition increase the risk for DM. Additionally, some data link increased leptin levels with diabetes.

<u>Benefits of controlling diabetes</u>

There are many benefits to controlling diabetes in the older population. First, there is the prevention of acute complications such as coma, ketoacidosis, and osmotic diuresis, which leads to dehydration. Additionally, there may be changes to vision, which may present a safety issue. Certain complications of diabetes such as peripheral vascular disease, retinopathy, and diabetic nephropathy may worsen if sufficient preventative measures are not taken. Foot complications may occur and can lead to amputation. Poor control of diabetes may also lead to impaired cognitive function and less favorable outcome following a stroke. Risk of heart attack is also increased.

<u>Factors that influence the decision to use insulin to treat diabetes</u>

Insulin therapy should be initiated if attempts at controlling diabetes with a combination of diet, exercise and oral agents have not been effective. Also, individuals with severe liver or renal dysfunction may have limited choices available to them for controlling blood glucose levels. Factors that should also be considered include the visual acuity level of the individual, the function of the hands and fingers, mental status, and finances. There are premixed insulin products available that will eliminate the need for patient mixing. There are also insulin syringes and pens with pre-measured doses that may be used to simplify an insulin regimen. Pens are often a safer choice for elderly adults. If regular syringes are used, the smallest applicable size should be employed to guard against mistakes and overdosing. Devices are available that attach to the syringe in order to magnify the labels to help with visibility.

<u>Treatment</u>

Treating diabetes mellitus in the geriatric population is a complicated science. Each treatment plan must be individualized and should be made in consideration of other chronic diseases, medication schedules, living situation, cognitive function, and overall life expectancy. Frail elders would not undergo the same rigorous treatment plan involving medication, increasing physical activity and dietary modifications that a healthier and more active elderly adult would. The main treatment goal is to control blood glucose levels but the level of control must be weighed against the risks and benefits of tight control. An acute hypoglycemic episode may be far more harmful than the cumulative effects of hyperglycemia. For example, even a slightly low blood glucose level may lead to a fall in an elderly adult, and this, in turn, may lead to a decline in functional status.

According to the American Diabetes Association, dietary management for a diabetic patient should be individualized and calories provided at a level that will help the person achieve and maintain an appropriate body weight. If weight loss is required, 10-20 pounds may have very positive effects on blood glucose control, reducing lipids and blood pressure, all of which improve overall health. Fat intake should be limited to approximately 30% of total calories with monounsaturated and polyunsaturated fats making up majority of those calories. Protein should contribute 10-20% of total calories to provide the recommended daily allowance of 0.8 grams per kg. The remainder of caloric intake should come from carbohydrates, preferably complex carbohydrates. Moreover, 20-35 grams per day fiber (soluble and insoluble) is the goal for most adults. For a frail elder or an elder living in a long-term care home, the risk for malnutrition is greater than the risk for developing complications from diabetes. Dietary modifications should be liberalized and the focus should be on consistent carbohydrate intake and prevention of malnutrition.

**HIV**

The incidence of HIV infection in elderly adults is estimated to be 15-20%. Moreover, the incidence of AIDS in this age group is rising more rapidly than in younger adults. Many professionals mistakenly believe that elderly adults are not at as great a risk for HIV as other age groups. However, elderly adults continue to be sexually active later in life, and often times, condoms are not used due to a lessened fear of pregnancy and/or knowledge and concern for prevention of sexually transmitted diseases.

Nutrition is one of the cornerstones of treatment for individuals with HIV infection. Consuming adequate calories helps with weight maintenance, and the prevention of wasting is imperative. Eating adequate amounts of protein, carbohydrate and fat is important to maintaining health. Protein is important to maintain visceral protein stores and daily requirements may range from 1-1.4 gm/kg for maintenance up to 2 gm/kg for repletion. Tolerance to fat may vary depending upon abdominal symptoms. Drinking plenty of fluids is essential to maintaining hydration and counteracting medication side effects. A daily multivitamin is often recommended. Food safety guidelines should be closely followed in order to reduce the risk of foodborne illness. Consultation with a registered dietician is recommended upon diagnosis of HIV and for any change in nutritional status.

## Special nutrition considerations

Age should not be the sole determinant in whether an individual should undergo surgical intervention. Preoperatively, any elderly surgical candidate should receive a full medical evaluation. The management of any pre-existing conditions, such as diabetes or heart disease, should be fully optimized before surgery. This would also include weight loss for those individuals who are to receive any type of orthopedic surgery, such as hip or knee replacement. Certain cases, such as fractured hip requiring immediate surgery, do not allow for this optimization of health. In this type of case, mortality is often higher. Screening for malnutrition is also important. Malnourished geriatric patients are at higher risk for developing nosocomial infections and pressure sores. Malnutrition also may lead to poor healing post-operatively, may increase the chance of surgical complications and prolong recovery time.  In some cases, the use of a preoperative tube feeding is useful in improving nutritional status.

# Nutrition Counseling And Education

**NCEP**

The National Heart, Blood and Lung Institute (NHBLI), which is part of the Department of Health and Human Services and the National Institute of Health initiated the National Cholesterol Education Program (NCEP) in 1985. The goal of the program was to reduce the incidence of cardiovascular disease by focusing on reducing cholesterol levels in Americans. The program is geared towards health professionals, the public and community. The Expert Panel on Detection, Evaluation and Treatment of High Blood Cholesterol in Adults issued its third report of the NCEP guidelines, and this report is referred to as the Adult Treatment Panel III or ATP III. The most important feature of ATP III is the challenge to more aggressively target individuals who have multiple cardiac risk factors.

The NCEP ATP (Adult Treatment Panel) guidelines encourage therapeutic lifestyle changes (TLC). These guidelines recommend that 25-35% of total calories come from fat, with less than 7% from saturated fat, 10% from polyunsaturated fat and up to 20% from monounsaturated fat. The guidelines also recommend 50-60% of total calories from carbohydrate, and 15% of total calories from protein. Dietary cholesterol should be less than 200 mg per day. Total calorie intake should be sufficient to achieve and maintain an ideal body weight while preventing weight gain. The ATP guidelines also recommend the addition of 2 grams per day of plant sterols/stanols and 10-25 grams per day of soluble fiber. These guidelines are geared towards individuals whose LDL cholesterol levels are greater than the goal LDL for their category of risk. This level of risk may be calculated using the National Heart, Blood, and Lung Institute's (NHBLI) ten-year risk calculator, which may be found on the NHBLI website.

The National Heart, Blood and Lung Institute (NHBLI), which is part of the Department of Health and Human Services and the National Institute of Health, initiated the National Cholesterol Education Program (NCEP) in 1985. The goal of the program was to reduce the incidence of cardiovascular disease by focusing on reducing cholesterol levels in Americans. The program is geared towards health professionals, the public and community. The Expert Panel on Detection, Evaluation and Treatment of High Blood Cholesterol in Adults issued its third report of the NCEP guidelines, and this report is referred to as the Adult Treatment Panel III or ATP III. The most important feature of ATP III is the challenge to more aggressively target individuals who have multiple cardiac risk factors.

**AHA versus ATP**

Previously, the American Heart Association's (AHA) guidelines included the Step I and II diets. These terms are no longer used. The new guidelines emphasize a diet low in both saturated and trans fat, promote the inclusion of whole grains, fresh fruits and vegetables, and recommend increasing one's consumption of fish. The AHA encourages restricting sodium intake to less than 2300 mg per day. The AHA now uses the therapeutic lifestyle changes (TLC) diet for those at high risk for cardiac disease. The TLC diet essentially replaced the Step II AHA diet. Both the ATP III and AHA continue to recommend guidelines similar to what was traditionally recommended in the AHA Step I diet. This includes limiting fat intake to 30% of total calories, restricting saturated fat to less than 10% of calories, and limiting total dietary cholesterol to less than 300 mg per day.

**Calcium and uric acid stones**

Renal changes, such as those affecting the concentration of urine or pH, may lead to the formation of kidney stones. The two most common types of kidney stones are calcium and uric acid stones. Calcium stones are due to hypercalciuria, and this may be caused by a defect in calcium absorption, a change in renal function, increased calcium losses due to immobility, or hypercalcemia resulting from another cause. Generally, individuals with normal serum calcium but with hypercalciuria are encouraged to increase fluid intake to more than two liters per day while restricting intake of high calcium foods, such as dairy products. Uric acid stones may require limitation of protein containing foods. Allopurinol is generally prescribed to treat these stones and would make diet restrictions unnecessary

## Change model stages

The stages of change model are a process that individuals go through in order to achieve behavioral change. There are six steps that have been identified. The first three are as follows:

1. *Precontemplation:* This stage occurs before an individual has even considered making a change in behavior.

2. *Contemplation:* This stage occurs once the individual is aware of the problem that needs to be addressed but experiences a period where advantages and disadvantages are weighed carefully.

3. *Preparation:* This is the stage where the individual will either move forward or revert back to the contemplation stage. The individual requires assistance in identifying action steps or establishing goals to make the overall change achievable.

4. *Action:* This stage is where the steps that need to be taken are implemented in order to affect change.

5. *Maintenance:* This stage involves continued behavior modification and determination to influence change prevent relapse to old habits.

- 108 -

6.  *Relapse:* This stage may occur if the individual reverts to old behavior. It is not uncommon for patients to revert, and therefore, revisit the action stage.

It is beneficial for a registered dietician (RD) and/or nutrition educator to know what stage of change an individual is in because it allows the professional to the ability to more effectively plan teaching strategies. When RD's are trying to perform nutrition education, many individuals begin in a stage where they are not yet ready to make change, which will contribute to lack of success. Knowing the stages of change assists, allows professionals the ability to move clients productively towards change.

## Adult learners

Adults learn differently than children and adolescents. Adult learners are autonomous and self-directed. They want to be actively involved in the learning process and often learn best when they assume some of this responsibility. Adults have a large base of life experiences and prior knowledge. Drawing on this base and relating the information being taught to this base is important. Adults are also goal-oriented and want to be able to find a way to achieve the goals they have set for themselves. Adults also need motivation for learning. Educational content must be applicable to their life, their health or their work. Practicality of material is highly desirable to adult learners. The lesson being taught must be applicable, at least in part, to some other aspect of the individual's life. Adults also need to be treated with respect in terms of the knowledge and experience they possess.

## Learning and changing barriers

There are many barriers to learning in the elderly adult population. These barriers may include other responsibilities, such as taking care of a sick spouse or time constraints. Other barriers include financial constraints, lack of confidence or motivation, transportation issues, and health issues. Literacy levels and cultural factors will also play a role in one's ability to learn. Ageism is another barrier in that there may be a belief that change may not be affected beyond a certain age. It may also be the belief that elderly adults are set in their ways and are thus unable to change or that health will not be improved. Individual barriers include adequacy of sight and hearing, mobility, chewing and swallowing difficulties, level of alertness and memory status. Another barrier to change is fear of or resistance to technology if advanced types of technology are used.

## Promoting dietary changes

There are quite a few ways to promote health related changes to an elderly adult. These include effective educational strategies. Lessons may be better received if they include videos, presentations by an expert or a peer with relating experience, demonstrations, and printed materials. Mentors, small group discussions, and/or peer exchanges regarding the topic may also promote change. One on one counseling is also an option. The educator needs to help the learner acquire the information needed to make informed decisions. Barriers should be identified and addressed by the educator. A social and emotional support system should be identified to encourage change. Coping strategies and problem solving skills should be taught. Concrete suggestions for ways to modify behavior are helpful. Providing positive suggestions, such as what to eat, rather than negative instruction, such as what not to eat, is generally more productive. Ultimately the client must know, understand, and agree with the reason for dietary modification if change is desired.

## Improving communication

Health care professionals should always ensure that they are effectively communicating with their patients. Factors to consider in communication include assessing sensory losses that may affect communication and ensuring assistive devices, such as glasses or hearing aids, are in place and functioning. For those with impaired hearing, speak slowly and carefully while facing the individual to allow full view of lips. Distracting noises should be eliminated and one should speak loudly and clearly while being careful to maintain normal pitch. Eye contact should be maintained. Rooms should be well lit to help those with impaired sight, and glare should be minimized. Yes or no questions should be asked if the individual is aphasic. The individual's mental status should be assessed especially if confusion is apparent. The professional should attempt communicating with the patient at his/her best time of day. Gentle touch is often useful in communicating with elderly adults. Non-verbal cues by the professional will reflect the level of care and compassion.

## Developing nutrition education

When developing nutrition education materials targeted for elderly adults, there are several factors to consider. First, materials should be designed simply, and there should be a sharp contrast between the color of the text and the background color. A large font size should be used fancy type fonts avoided. Margins and line spacing should be large. Sensitivity to religious and cultural issues should always be maintained. Low literacy levels should be addressed using plain language. The information presented should be of value to the targeted population and the information should be easy to use. The number of messages presented should be limited to four ideas or less. Specific action steps and recommendations for making changes should be provided.

## Lowering sodium

The most frequently used and problematic source of dietary sodium is the salt shaker and it should be avoided. Processed foods, such as cured meats (ham, bacon, hot dogs, sausages, etc.) and cured fish (anchovies, sardines, etc.), are the second most sodium-loaded consumables. Canned soups and vegetables should be avoided unless they have reduced sodium content. Snack foods, such as chips, pretzels, popcorn and various types of crackers with salted tops, should also be avoided. Additionally, prepared sauces and condiments, such as certain salad dressings, relish, mustard, ketchup, soy sauce, barbecue sauce and gravies should be avoided on a low-sodium diet. Frozen dinners should be avoided and if this is a regular part of an elderly adult's diet, alternative meals need to be identified. Processed cheeses such as prepackaged slices and spreads contain significant amounts of sodium and should be avoided. Reading nutrition labels is an important component of achieving a low sodium diet. Nutrition counseling with a registered dietician should be arranged to help ensure success.

# Nutrition Monitoring And Evaluation

## Monitoring CHD patients

An individual who has started the TLC (therapeutic lifestyle changes) diet should be reducing saturated fat and cholesterol in their diet as well as increasing physical activity. A referral to a registered dietician is beneficial. After six weeks, the individual's LDL cholesterol level should be reevaluated. If the level is not at the previously determined goal, additional measures should be instituted. This may include the addition of plant stanols/sterols, increasing soluble fiber intake and the provision of additional support for implementing dietary changes. This plan should be reevaluated again after another six weeks. If the LDL level has not been reduced to the optimal level specified, drug therapy should be considered.

## Evaluation process

The risks and benefits of any type of dietary restriction in an elderly adult should be fully evaluated prior to initiation of such restrictions. Implementation of any restriction should also be fully evaluated for feasibility. Many elderly individuals have low caloric intake, and the quality of one's diet is associated with caloric intake. Restricting food intake further may lead to nutrient deficiencies. An increase in physical activity without reducing caloric intake may be one way to address an elevated BMI. Any dietary restrictions or modifications should be made in conjunction with the individual in order to integrate religious and cultural preferences. The registered dietician (RD) should work closely with the patient to education him/her regarding appropriate food choices for specialized diets. For example, if an elderly man needs to reduce sodium intake but frequently consumes frozen meals; the RD must education the patient as to his easy to prepare alternatives. Education and assistance will greatly improve the patient's ability to achieve dietary goals where compliance is otherwise unlikely.

## Cholesterol-reducing drug therapy

Drug therapy is generally started based on level of cardiac risk. A category I risk is defined as an individual who already has heart disease, diabetes and other risk factors, and in this case, the goal LDL cholesterol level is less than 100 mg/dl. Category I patients are started on drug therapy immediately.

Patients in other risk categories may be able to wait three months before discussing drug therapy depending upon overall cardiac risk. The waiting period will allow the healthcare professional to determine if lifestyle changes have been effective in lowering LDL cholesterol. If an individual falls into Category II, which is the second highest risk level, and has an LDL greater than 130 mg/dl; he/she may need immediate drug therapy. If an individual falls into Category III, which indicates moderate risk, with an LDL level greater than 160 mg/dl, drugs are initiated immediately. Finally, an individual who falls in Category IV, which indicates low to moderate risk, LDL levels greater than 160 mg/dl after three months of therapeutic lifestyle changes (TLC) would indicate the need for drug therapy.

## Blood glucose control

Hemoglobin A1c levels less than 7% indicate healthy blood glucose in elderly adults who have fairly good health and are independent. The actual goal for glucose control should be individualized based on functional status, life expectancy, and the presence of other chronic conditions. Any elderly individual who has a blood glucose level less than 100 mg/dl requires further evaluation. A history should be taken to determine if the individual is eating, needs assistance with meal preparation, is experiencing an increase in the frequency of falls, etc.

Many elderly adults may not be as astute at recognizing the symptoms of hypoglycemia and the symptoms may actually be milder in elderly adults.

Generally speaking, blood glucose control in elderly inpatients falls somewhere between preventing hypoglycemia and the metabolic effects of hypoglycemia, such as dehydration. In other words, many hospitals take a minimalist approach to blood glucose control in inpatients. Recent studies suggest, however, that a more proactive approach to diabetes control for inpatients may reduce morbidity and mortality in ICU patients, patients waiting for surgery and those recovering from a heart attack.

## Evidence-based Nutrition Practice Guidelines

Evidence-based Nutrition Practice Guidelines were developed by the American Dietetic Association and are used as an algorithm for treating various disease states. They assist the registered dietician in analyzing and synthesizing data, which in turn, leads to more appropriate decisions regarding nutrition care. As of 2008, the following adult guidelines were available: adult weight management, critical illness, disorders of lipid metabolism, and oncology. Information is separated into the following categories: introduction, major recommendations, algorithms, background information, appendices and reference list. For example, the adult weight management module deals with nutrition assessment and treatment including classification of BMI, weight management programs and program duration. It also includes dietary interventions such as reduced calorie diets and education. Other topics include special dietary approaches, such as a low glycemic index diet or low carbohydrate diets. The guidelines include physical activity recommendations and behavior management strategies. Finally, the guidelines cover medications and bariatric surgery.

## Administration on Aging

Many nutrition programs administered by the Administration on Aging (AoA) and the Older Americans Act (OAA) have favorable outcomes. One goal of the programs is to increase the number of participants served each year and to target isolated and vulnerable elderly individuals. Another goal is to continue to provide high quality service. This goal is measured through participant satisfaction with home delivered or congregate meals. Another outcome measure for this goal is caregiver satisfaction and the ability of a participant to stay in his/her home past previous expectations. An additional goal is to reduce the number of participants who have difficulty acquiring services. Moreover, the program aims to improve nutritional intake of elderly adults who receive home delivered or congregate meals. Outcome measures for this goal would include self-reported data on nutritional adequacy of the participant's diet and the ability to maintain a specialized diet, such as reduced sodium or fat diet.

## Monitoring and evaluation

The nutrition monitoring and evaluation part of the nutrition care process is a valuable step in assessing the effectiveness of the nutrition intervention. The monitoring piece refers to reviewing available data and comparing data to the plan, expected outcomes and goals. The evaluation piece involves comparing data to previous patient status or a reference standard. For example, if the goal was to lower cholesterol level, then initial serum cholesterol levels should be compared to levels following the intervention phase. The overall purpose of this step is to see if progress is being made toward achieving established goals. Methods of information collection include reviewing data entered in the medical record, monitoring height and weight, and compilation of other anthropometric data. Obtaining the information necessary to complete this phase of the nutrition care process may be challenging, and thus, creative methods of acquiring the data may be necessary. Some methods may include making phone calls or sending reminder postcards to the patients.

## Nutrition intervention outcomes

The outcomes should be concrete goals that are directly related to the nutrition diagnosis. Examples of outcomes may be amount of knowledge gained or retained changes in behavior, improvement in nutritional status, or changes in laboratory values. It may also include changes in clinical condition such as improvement in blood pressure, blood glucose control, weight, reduction of risk factors, reduction in symptoms, or improvement in overall clinical status. Outcomes may be health-centered or centered around an individuals wellbeing such that improvement in quality of life, the ability to care for oneself, or the ability to be self-sufficient may be included. Other types of measurable outcomes include change in medication, reduction of health care costs, reduction in visits to the clinic, fewer admissions to the hospital, or delayed admission to a skilled nursing facility. It may be useful to evaluate progress towards a goal using a numerical scale, such as a range of 1-5. Other appropriate types of reference standards may be utilized.

## Continuing nutrition services

There are several points during the nutrition care process where the determination for continuing nutrition services may be made. The first is after the assessment/reassessment of the patient. The registered dietician (RD) may determine that nutritional care will not be of further assistance in addressing an individual's nutrition issues, and the individual may be discharged from nutritional care. The second point at which a determination regarding the continuation of nutritional services occurs after nutrition intervention. At this time, the RD determines whether the individual has met the established goals. The RD may also evaluate the individual's willingness to make appropriate changes at that time. Discharge from nutrition care would be appropriate if the patient is unwilling to attempt necessary dietary changes. The last point in the nutrition care process that the need for continued nutrition care services is considered is during the monitoring and evaluation step. The outcomes of the attempted nutritional therapy will be evaluated and will aid the RD in determining whether to continue care.

## PEG tube complications

There are many potential complications of PEG (percutaneous endoscopic gastrostomy) tubes. These complications can impact a patient's quality of life by causing additional pain and suffering. The complications may include localized pain or bleeding at the insertion site, cellulitis, or abdominal wall abscess. Mechanical complications may include problems with the tube such as leakage, obstruction or becoming dislodged. Gastrointestinal complications may include nausea, vomiting, changes in bowel function, reflux, bowel obstruction, or gastrointestinal bleeding. Some gastrointestinal complications may necessitate surgical intervention, which will add to pain and suffering. Fever and sepsis are possible. Aspiration pneumonia is also a potential complication. Other complications may include loss of ability to feed orally, changes in social function, changes in metabolic status, or fluid overload.

# Food Services

### Dining program in nursing homes

The availability of adequate, meal-time assistance has been identified as an essential factor in preventing malnutrition in nursing homes. Therefore, it is important that all facilities develop a comprehensive dining program. The first step to program development is appointing a dining coordinator. This person is responsible for the overall function of the dining room, including staffing of the personnel who may assist residents with meals, training, procedural development, and implementation of the program. The next step to program formation is to evaluate the needs of each resident in terms of assistance required at meals. Staffing needs are determined next; and they may range from one staff member per eight residents to one staff member to every two residents requiring complete assistance. Next, the procedure must be implemented. This includes training staff members in topics, such as proper positioning, adaptive utensils, and recognizing swallowing issues. Finally, ongoing evaluation is important to any dining program. Evaluation should include reassessment of resident needs every 3-6 months or as necessary, evaluation of staffing levels, and safety issues.

### CACFP

The CACFP (Child and Adult Care Food Program) is a federal program, sponsored by the United States Department of Agriculture (USDA) and administered at the state level, which reimburses centers that provide meals to elderly and/or functionally impaired adults. It also reimburses centers for meals served to certain populations of children. Centers qualifying for reimbursements include licensed adult day programs operated by non-profit organizations and certain for-profit organizations if they serve the targeted population (elderly and/or disabled individuals). Reimbursements are dependent upon the number of free or reduced-cost meals and snacks provided to targeted populations. Specific meal patterns are provided and must be met as a condition of reimbursement. For example, a lunch pattern for an adult consists of one cup of milk, two cups of fruits/vegetables, one serving of grain product, and one meat or meat alternative. Portion sizes and alternative suggestions are provided in order to assist centers in meeting reimbursement requirements.

**Food safety issues**

It is important that elderly adults are educated in regards to proper food safety. As an individual ages, the effect of food poisoning may be exacerbated, and often times, elderly adults take longer to recover from these types of illnesses. Age- and medication-related changes in taste or smell may make it more difficult for elderly patients to discern whether food is spoiled. Refrigerated foods should be maintained at or below 40 °F and freezer foods at or below 0 °F. Proper thawing of meat is essential, and good hand washing is important, especially after touching raw meats. Cutting surfaces should be sanitized with a bleach solution. It is important to impart the danger of consuming foods in the danger zone of 40-140 °F. Food should not stay out longer than two hours. This includes home delivered meals. These should be consumed within two hours or properly stored for future use.

**Menu planning**

The Older Americans Act (OAA) stipulates that nutrition programs serving elderly adults must meet the Dietary Guidelines for Americans and must provide at least 1/3 of the dietary reference intakes for elderly adults. Registered dietitians (RD) should be available to assist with menu planning and meal pattern development. Ideally, menu input should be obtained from the clients as well as the food production staff. Nutrient analysis software is an excellent tool to use for assistance with menu planning. Some programs analyze recipes as well as track production, inventory, cost analysis, and other needs. Specialized diets complicate the process somewhat but must be addressed. Texture modified diets must be taken into account, planned and prepared under the guidance of a RD and speech pathologist or occupational therapist.

## Ethnic and religious needs

Nutrition programs must be designed such that religious and ethnic preferences are incorporated and observed. Some ethnic foods, such as spaghetti and meatballs, corned beef and cabbage, and fried chicken are standard meal options for many programs. Suggestions for planning an ethnically or religiously diverse menu include soliciting opinions from a diverse sampling of clients, families, and communities. Additionally, employing staff members who are culturally diverse may encourage menu diversity as well. Invite guest chefs who are experienced in preparing diverse food to visit and cook for the program on a regular basis. As the established meal pattern allows, ask an ethnic caterer or restaurant to provide meals to the program. New foods may be introduced around religious or ethnic holidays.

## Safety and sanitation requirements

Programs that provide meals for elderly adults must meet all safety and sanitation requirements set by federal, state and local agencies. If part of the program is contracted out, the contractor must also meet all the requirements. All service providers must conform to standards set by local boards of health. Food temperature is of utmost concern and care must be taken to keep all foods out of the danger zone of 40-140 ° F. Thermometers must be used to monitor food temperatures and must also be used in refrigerators and freezers to maintain appropriate temperatures. Equipment should meet the requirements of the National Sanitation Foundation or of state and local health departments. All fire and safety codes must also be obeyed and regular inspections need to be conducted to ensure compliance.

**Training personnel**

Minimum standards have been set for programs administered through the Older Americans Act (OAA), and these include personnel training. Training is essential in order to address the changing needs of the population, improve outcomes, incorporate research into practice, promote innovative procedures and ensure skill levels are kept up-to-date. Factors influencing training include the size of the program, funding level, type of population served, and the program's goals and objectives. Other factors include the education, skill and knowledge level of personnel. The cost of the program, access to material or technology, location of training, commitment of personnel and managers, and expected outcomes are additional factors to take into account. High turnover of personnel may greatly affect training issues.

Training methods vary greatly. Traditional methods, such as books, newsletters or lectures, remain important as technological skill levels among personnel may vary. The use of television and videotapes are also an option. Technological methods that are available include the use of CR-ROMs or the Internet to access websites, such as the National Institute on Aging or the Administration on Aging, for information. Interactive training methods may include videoconferencing or interactive stations set up at senior centers. Personnel should also receive training that teaches them how to teach clients to use technological tools that may be used during assessments.

## Preparing elderly for disasters

Planning for disasters is essential. In addition to having a first aid kit, an extra supply of prescription drugs, important papers, and emergency contact numbers, elderly individuals must have adequate food and water stores available. One gallon of water per person per day, with provisions for at least three days, is recommended. Elderly individuals should be encouraged to have additional water supply as dehydration is dangerous. Water should be kept in small, easy-to-open containers, which are more manageable to handle are more suitable to arthritic hands. At least a three day supply of food is recommended. Food stores must take into account special dietary needs. Manual can openers and other essential tools should also be included in the emergency supply kit.

## OBRA

The 1987 OBRA (Omnibus Reconciliation Act) legislation set minimum nutritional care and dietary service staffing standards. Nursing homes accepting Medicaid reimbursement must employ a registered dietician as either a permanent employee or consultant. Additionally, the facility must employ enough staff to carry out food service functions. Menus must meet dietary reference intakes, and food must be palatable and served at appropriate temperatures. If a resident refuses a meal, a substitute of equal nutritional value must be offered. Three meals per day, at minimum, must be served, and fourteen hours is the maximum time allowed between dinner and breakfast unless a substantial evening snack is provided. In this case, sixteen hours between meals is allowed. Assistive devices must be available for residents who require them. Physician must prescribe therapeutic diets. Standards for weight loss specifying when intervention should occur are also included in the act.

## Dementia patients

Individuals with dementia may experience an array of issues that can affect mealtime and eating. Some of those issues and coping methods are listed below;

- *Forgetfulness:* A simple, structured routine is important. Coping methods also include seating the patient in the same place each meal, limiting his/her choices, and removing distractions.
- *Paranoia:* A simple, structured routine is also helpful in this situation. Medications should not be hidden in food as this may exacerbate symptoms of paranoia. Serving foods in containers with lids is recommended.
- *Inability to concentrate:* The individual should be guided through the meal gentle words. Food and beverage should be in sight and utensils positioned in the hands.
- *Unwillingness to attend the meal service:* Meals may be served in the individual's room or at another location; however, the person should be questioned about his/her reluctance to eat in the dining room. One-on-one meals may be more comfortable to the patient than a group setting.

Dementia patients may struggle to complete meals. Below are some common problems encountered by dementia patients at mealtime and mechanisms for coping with those challenges.

- *Consumes meals too quickly:* Food items should be offered separately. Offer foods that require more chewing, if patient is able to safely and effectively chew. A smaller spoon or fork may be useful. Provide verbal cues to slow down while eating.
- *Consuming meals too slowly:* Verbally coax the patient to continue eating and taking bites. This individual should be served first to allow additional time to eat.

- *Forgets to swallow:* Verbal reminders to swallow throughout the meal are necessary to prevent pocketing the food. Monitor the swallow by feeling and/or coax the swallow by lightly rubbing the larynx.
- Chews endlessly: If the individual chews without swallowing, he/she will need verbal reinforcement after each bite to initiate the swallow. Softer foods and smaller bites may also be helpful.

The following are behaviors exhibited by dementia patients. Each behavior is followed by coping strategies.

- *Frequent spitting:* A chewing and swallow evaluation should be completed. Seat the patient away from others who may be bothered by this behavior. Remind the patient that spitting is inappropriate.
- *Combative behavior:* Position the staff aide on the patient's weak (non-dominant) side. Use unbreakable tableware. Reward appropriate behavior.
- *Plays with food:* Offer only one food at a time. Serve food in small portions and cover it when appropriate. Offer finger foods.

# Professional Practices

## Title III and VI ENP

Title III and VI Elder Nutrition Program (ENP) is a federal program funded by the Department of Health and Human Services Administration on Aging and Office of Human Development Services. ENP was introduced as an amendment to the Older American Acts of 1965. It is the largest federally-funded and most comprehensive program involving community and home care services that benefit the geriatric population. The program provides at least one meal per day, at least five days per week. Moreover, the program supplies at least one third of the recommended daily allowance. ENP provides congregate meals as well as home delivered meals. ENP also includes access initiatives that include transportation services, in-home services such as home health aides, and community based health and social services such as case management, fitness programs, etc. ENP serves adults over the age of 60 and their spouses. Payment for services is completely voluntary.

The ENP is a major benefit to elderly adults and is not dependent upon income level, social situation, or health status. The ENP provides regular socialization to many elderly adults who may not otherwise have such an opportunity. ENP programs also provide at least one nutritious meal per day to participants to prevent malnutrition. Additionally, the programs address health issues impacted by food and nutrition. ENP also provides nutrition screening to identify elderly adults at risk for malnutrition. Nutritional counseling and education are provided as needed. This program also allows elderly adults to maintain independence in their homes for as long as possible. The programs are often placed in low income areas to make ENP more accessible to elderly participants. Contributions to ENP programs are strictly voluntary.

**Food Stamp program**

The Food Stamp Program is a program administered by the United States Department of Agriculture. It is a program that provides income assistance in the form of coupons or electronic benefit transfer (EBT) cards for the purpose of purchasing food. The benefit of the EBT card is that the cash value is automatically reloaded each month eliminating the need to visit the food stamp office for benefits. The amount of assistance received is based on income and other factors. The criteria are slightly different for adults over sixty and the disabled population than for other populations. Benefits may be administered even if the beneficiary possesses some cash assets. The coupons or EBT cards may be used at supermarkets and many other places where food is sold. Food Stamps may only be used to purchase food and not alcohol, tobacco or other non-food items.

Participation rates among elderly adults are low for the Food Stamp program. Less than 10% of all participants are over the age of sixty. Many elderly individuals are reluctant to participate due to the stigma of accepting government handouts associated with the Food Stamp Program. Additionally, individuals often falsely believe that the application process is cumbersome. Another barrier may be the electronic benefit transfer (EBT) cards that are used, as many elderly individuals are not accustomed to using this type of technology. Congress has implemented provisions to address the low participation rates of seniors by making applications available at Social Security offices, providing assistance with the application process to those who receive Social Security Supplemental Income (SSI), and allowing coupons to be used at certain restaurants. The in-office interview requirement is waived for elderly individuals. A number of outreach programs have also been implemented to try to reach this population.

## Purpose of Medicare

Medicare is a national insurance program for individuals over the age of 65 and for individuals younger than 65 who have kidney failure or other specified disabilities. It is administered by the Centers for Medicare and Medicaid Services (CMS) and was originally developed under the 1965 Social Security Act. The Medicare program has partnerships with many hospitals, nursing homes, physicians, HMOs, suppliers of medical equipment, and numerous other services associated with healthcare. Medicare provides third party reimbursement for health-related expenses, insurance for hospitalization and long term care benefits for all eligible individuals. There are two parts to Medicare: Part A and B. Over 40 million individuals over the age of 65 receive Medicare benefits.

## Medicare covered Diabetes services

The following services are covered in part or fully by Medicare:

- *Diabetes screening:* Up to two screenings per year for individuals over the age of 65, who are overweight, or have risk factors for diabetes.
- *Diabetes Self-Management Training:* Available with a written, physician's order. Allows patient a pre-specified number of visits to a certified program.
- *Diabetes supplies and services:* Supplies such as syringes, lancets, blood glucose test strips and monitors are covered. Insulin is covered under the prescription drug program.
- *Medical Nutrition Therapy:* Covered with a physician order. Must be provided by a registered dietician or Medicare-approved professional.
- *Foot exams:* Covered for patients with diabetes-related peripheral neuropathy. Therapeutic shoes and inserts are also covered for those with diabetes-related foot conditions.

## Covered under Medicare Part A

Medicare Part A covers many of the costs of care associated with hospitalization and skilled nursing facilities. The individual must pay co-insurance and deductibles. Part A covers a semi-private hospital room, board, nursing, therapies, medications, supplies, laboratory tests, radiology, intensive care, operating rooms and any other service deemed medically necessary. Medicare does not pay for any extraneous and optional services, such as television, private rooms or private duty nurses. In a skilled nursing facility, a semi-private room is covered as well as meals, skilled nursing services and rehabilitative therapies such as physical or occupational therapy. Coverage is defined by length of stay. Days 1-20 are covered in full, while days 21 -100 are prorated, and coverage ends after 100 days. Part A also covers home health services, such as some nursing care, home health aides, and certain durable medical equipment. Hospice care is also covered if prescribed by a physician.

## Covered under Medicare Part B

Medicare Part B is considered to be the medical insurance portion of Medicare. Medicare approved physicians, facilities and other service providers must be utilized. It is generally responsible for the payment of any outpatient service. Covered medical expenses include physician visits, therapies such as physical, occupational or speech, mental health services, durable medical equipment and medical supplies. It also helps cover ambulance services. Preventive care is also included, such as flu shots or mammograms. Part B will cover home health services if the individual does not have Medicare Part A. Part B will cover some medical services not covered by Part A. medical nutrition therapy is covered under part B and is discussed in detail on another flashcard.

## JCAHO

JCAHO is an organization that provides voluntary inspections of healthcare facilities and sets standards of care that must be met to attain accreditation. Nutrition services that are mandated as part of the accreditation process include nutrition screening and assessment, diet counseling, and provision of clinical nutrition care such as enteral and parenteral nutrition therapy. Nutrition screening is an especially integral part of the accreditation process as JCAHO recognizes the impact of malnutrition on hospital outcome. It also provides guidelines for the operation of food service systems, including sanitation standards and provision of therapeutic diets. As part of the accreditation process, qualified nutrition professionals make up the healthcare team that provides clinical nutrition services and food services. Documentation of appropriate training and education is required.

## TEFAP

TEFAP (The Emergency Food Assistance Program) is a federal food assistance program that provides food in bulk to the nation's food banks. The food banks then distribute the food to food pantries and soup kitchens. Funding comes from the Farm Bill, which also provides money for the Senior Farmer's Market Nutrition Program and the Fresh Fruit and Vegetable Program. The amount of food each state receives is dependent upon the size of the unemployed and low income populations of the state. The criterion for eligibility is determined at the state level but is usually includes low income residents. Often times, beneficiaries receive additional types of aid. Distributed food includes a variety of canned fruits and vegetables, juices, dried beans, canned or frozen meats, rice, pasta, and cereals. Food may also be used to prepare congregate meals, such as those served at homeless shelters or senior centers.

**Medical Wavers**

Medicaid Waivers is a program that enables adults who are financially and medically qualified for participation in the Medicaid Nursing Home Program to remain in and receive care at their homes vice a nursing home or long-term care facility. Services that are provided include adult daycare, emergency response services, personal care, meal assistance and respite care. The program also provides skilled nursing care, home health aides, personal care assistants, and allows for home modifications. The goal of the program is to encourage independence for as long as possible. Financial eligibility differs from regular Medicaid coverage. An individual's income and assets are considered. Medically, the individual must meet the criteria for nursing home eligibility, including both physical and functional requirements.

**PACE**

PACE, Program of All-Inclusive Care for the Elderly, is a capitated program that incorporates service delivery with Medicaid and Medicare financing. This program was developed as part of the Balanced Budget Act of 1997, to address the needs of certain individuals, payers, and providers. The individuals must be over the age of 55, live in a PACE area, and meet eligibility requirements for nursing home care. The service part of the package allows for frail individuals to live at home and receive appropriate services rather than in a nursing facility. The program promotes independent living. The capitated piece of the program allows providers to deliver required services without worry whether Medicaid or Medicare will cover the services. PACE providers receive monthly capitation payments for each individual enrolled in the program.

**NSIP**

The Nutrition Services Incentive Program (NSIP) is a program that was originally authorized by the Older Americans Act (OAA) of 2000. The United States Department of Agriculture (USDA) initially administered it. In 2003, administration was transferred to the Administration on Aging (AoA), which is part of the Department of Health and Human Services. The purpose of the program was to create an incentive for the States Units on Aging (SUA) and Indian Tribal Organizations (ITO) to provide nutritious meals for elderly residents. These agencies receive cash or commodity grants in exchange for agreeing to participate in the program. There are many requirements that must be met in order for meals to qualify for reimbursement under the NSIP. For example, the agency serving the meal must have a contract with the SUA or ITO, the participant must be over the age of sixty, and the meal must meet the requirements of the OAA (Title III-C). Programs receiving Medicaid waivers are not eligible to participate.

**OAA Title III-C**

The OAA (Older Americans Act) was initially written in 1965, with the last amendment occurring in 2006. Title III-C is the section that addresses nutrition services. This part of the act authorizes congregate meals for the purpose of reducing hunger and food insecurity, providing socialization for elders and the promotion of good health by providing access to education and disease prevention services. It also authorizes one home delivered meal, at least five days per week. Title III-C also incorporates education and counseling as needed. The last part of Title III-C mandates that a registered dietician or someone with equivalent training be involved in the provisions f these services. Furthermore, meals must provide at least one-third of the recommended daily allowance of nutrients. Title III-C encourages joint participation with schools and similar institutions to promote intergenerational. The act further encourages program administration within close proximity to participant residences and limits the amount of time meals may be in transit before reaching participants.

## JCAHO abbreviations

In 2004, as part of the National Patient Safety Goals initiative a standardized list of "do not use" abbreviations, symbols and acronyms were identified and are as follows:

- *U:* Unit, but may be misinterpreted as 4 or 0. Unit should be spelled out.
- *IU:* International unit, but may be mistaken for 10 or IV (intravenous). International unit should be written out.
- *QD:* Every day, but there are many different ways to write this, such as Q.D. or qd. Daily should be written out.
- *Q.O.D.:* Every other day, but there are various ways to write this, which may cause confusion. Every other day should be written out.
- *Trailing zero:* (i.e., 2.0 mg) should be written as 2 mg
- *Missing lead zero:* (i.e., .2 mg) should be written as 0.2 mg
- *MS:* May indicate magnesium sulfate or morphine sulfate; $MgSO_4$ and $MSO_4$ may be confused with one another.

## International Classification of Diseases

Kwashiorkor malnutrition: 260.0

ICD-9-CM stands for International Classification of Diseases, 9th Revision, and Clinical Modifications. These are codes based on the World Health Organization ICD 9 codes and are used for assigning codes to procedures and diagnoses for reimbursement purposes. These codes were developed by the Centers for Medicare and Medicaid Services, the American Hospital Association, the American Health Information Management Association, and the National Center for Health Statistics. The use of these codes ensures consistency.

<u>261.0 marasmus and 263.0 malnutrition of moderate degree</u>

The criteria for code 261.0 indicating marasmus includes weight measure less than 80% of standard, a greater than 10% weight change during a six-month period, or both. Visceral protein stores are usually preserved as evidenced by serum albumin greater than 3 g/dl. Marasmus is caused by a chronic calorie deficiency, and fat and muscle catabolism are noticeable. Other characteristics include weakness and lethargy. The criteria for code 263.0, malnutrition of moderate degree, includes weight measuring between 60-75% of standard for height, and a mild depletion of visceral protein stores as evidenced by a serum albumin level between 3-3.5 g/dl.

<u>262.0 severe protein energy malnutrition and 263.1 malnutrition of mild degree</u>

The criteria for code 262.0, severe protein energy malnutrition (PEM), consists of a weight measure that is less than 60% of standard weight for height and depleted visceral protein stores, as evidenced by a serum albumin less than 3 g/dl. This type of malnutrition occurs when an individual with marasmus experiences additional physical stresses, such as surgery, infection or other acute illness. This type of PEM is a combination of marasmus and kwashiorkor. Such a combination results in high risk for infections and wound healing.

The criteria for code 263.1, malnutrition of mild degree, include a weight measure 60-75% of standard weight for height, and no significant depletion of visceral protein stores as evidenced by a serum albumin level of 3.5-5 g/dl.

## Legal terms

Living will, durable power of attorney for healthcare, and advanced directives:

- *Living will:* A legal document in which an individual specifies the type of care he/she wishes to receive in the event he/she becomes terminally ill and unable to speak for him/herself. Consultation with the primary care physician is helpful in order to ensure all options are discussed prior to drafting a living will it is also important to review these wishes in advance with family, close friends, and other trusted people, such as a member of the clergy.

- *Durable power of attorney for healthcare:* This is a legal document in which an individual appoints a representative (usually a family member or close friend) to make healthcare decisions for the individual in the event that he/she becomes incapacitated. The representative should be willing to act in accordance with the individual's wishes, even if the representative is not in agreement.

- *Advance directive:* A legal document that includes the above two components in order to provide guidance for making medical decisions. This may also specify wishes regarding tube feeding, hydration, and other end-of-life interventions.

## Tube feedings to sustain life

There are many ethical considerations regarding initiation of tube feedings for an individual with dementia. There is no guarantee that the tube feedings will improve the quality of life. Moreover, complications from tube placement may cause additional discomfort. Improvement in nutritional status is also not a guarantee. Once tube feedings are initiated, these individuals are often denied the pleasure of eating. Dementia usually takes away many of the small pleasures in life, such as recognizing loved ones or remembering favorite

- 135 -

hobbies. Eating and tasting flavors may be one of the few enjoyable aspects of a dementia patient's life. Many families consent to tube placement because of fears that the individual will starve to death. In end stage Alzheimer's disease, patients often refuse food, and death usually occurs in a matter of days or weeks. During this phase, endorphins released by the body provide a pleasurable, comfortable feeling in terminally ill individuals. Comfort care, such as ice chips or food, may be provided for pleasure only.

## OBRA

In 1987, Congress approved legislation (OBRA) which aimed to improve the quality of care provided by nursing homes that receive federal and state Medicaid reimbursements. The legislation included minimum standards of nursing home care and uniform standards for all nursing homes that accept Medicaid payments These standards include scheduled resident needs reassessments, which address social, physical and psychological issues. Additional provisions guard against resident abuse. . The legislation also includes mandatory training for nurse's aides. It includes residents' rights, such as the right to privacy, to be free from restraints, to have needs accommodated, and the right to refuse a transfer. The Centers for Medicare and Medicaid Services (CMS) has the right to close down a facility for substandard care or neglect. The legislation aspired to improve both patient quality of life and overall quality of care.

## Withholding nutritional support

A physician's decision to withhold or withdraw nutritional support is a very difficult one. Some physicians may find it unethical to withhold or withdraw nutrition or hydration; however, the decision is not solely up to the physician. Situations where this may be applicable include the following:

- The primary care goal is palliative care.

- Symptoms of fluid overload are exacerbating the medical condition and would be alleviated by withholding nutrition.
- End stage organ failure.
- Continuing nutrition would prolong death or cause suffering.
- If the disease or condition is diagnosed as fatal.
- If metastatic cancer or end stage AIDS is also present.
- If significant, severe and irreversible impairment is present following a stroke.
- If the patient considers his or her quality of life to be poor.

## Older Americans Act

The Older Americans Act (OAA) assists with provision and coordination of services for older Americans. There are many programs available that address food and nutrition issues, income, disabilities, and housing concerns. These programs may include Food Stamps, Meals on Wheels or congregate meal programs, Social Security and Supplemental Security Income (SSI), federal housing programs, heating assistance, transportation programs, home health services, such as personal care attendants or home health aides, and respite services for caregivers. Outreach services are also available. Local social services may assist qualifying individuals with application paperwork for many of these programs. Participation in any of the above services increases the likelihood of receiving optimal nutrition as resources, such as food, money and assistance with obtaining or preparing food, is available to participants.

# Special Report: Additional Bonus Material

Due to our efforts to try to keep this book to a manageable length, we've created a link that will give you access to all of your additional bonus material.

Please visit http://www.mo-media.com/nutrition/bonuses to access the information.